I0704347

Suffering "Long Covid"

Alleviating My L.C. Symptoms

While Trying To Kill It
JZ Murdock

What happened

What I experienced

What worked...for me

And, what really didn't

Cover wrapped photo "23354"

CDC Public Domain image

Alissa Eckert, MSMI; Dan Higgins, MAMS © 2020

Description: Transmission electron microscopic image of an isolate from the first U.S. case of COVID-19, formerly known as 2019-nCoV. The spherical viral particles, colorized blue, contain cross-section through the viral genome, seen as black dots.

Back Cover photo "23311"

CDC Public Domain image

Hannah A Bullock; Azaibi Tamin © 2020

This illustration, created at the Centers for Disease Control and Prevention (CDC), reveals ultrastructural morphology exhibited by coronaviruses. Note the spikes that adorn the outer surface of the virus, which impart the look of a corona surrounding the virion, when viewed electron microscopically. A novel coronavirus, named Severe Acute Respiratory Syndrome coronavirus 2 (SARS-CoV-2), was identified as the cause of an outbreak of respiratory illness first detected in Wuhan, China in 2019. The illness caused by this virus has been named coronavirus disease 2019 (COVID-19).

Cover by Marvin Hayes © 2022

https://www.redbubble.com/people/marvinhayes/

Published by LgN Productions

Table of Contents

Preface

I wrote this book because I could. Because I feel well enough now to write it. Because I've long had the skills and knowledge one needs to write a book. But, to tell the truth? For a while I was concerned I may never again function at the levels I used to. Or if I even could write another book. To put one together, to write it, to clean it up, to finish it. I've tried here to do the best I can, under sometimes difficult conditions.

[NOTE, January 2024 updates are in square brackets like this one. It was recently pointed out to me there were some grammatical errors in this book. The fundamental information is all correct, it's just some minor points that fell by the wayside in my initial editing of this book toward publication. I was deeper into Long Covid than I am now. My mind is much clearer and better able toward attention to detail. So I've now given it a going through and correcting any minor errors I found. Since I would be updating the manuscript, I felt I should add an update section for new findings. I'd been thinking about that through all of 2023 but I just couldn't bring myself to do it. This was a difficult book to write as I was revisiting some painful events and times. While I still have Long Covid, it's much slighter, flaring up from time to time and/or activating an underlying dormant viral infection. All this will be explained as you move through the book. For those who read the original version, thank you and I appreciate your understanding and patience. Cheers! Sláinte! (Gaelic for "On your Health!")]

This book has been delayed multiple times due to COVID-19 and Long Covid. I would preferred to have released it in 2020, or 2021. By 2022 I thought it might be too late. Or that I may not have anything to add to the discussion. On the other hand, in having waited, there was more research to draw upon. As for those worried about the correct or appropriate capitalization of

COVID in this book (as it had various iterations in the beginning of the pandemic)...I suspect we have far more important things to concern ourselves with here.

Then I caught it again. End of March, which led once again to Long Covid. I decided I finally had something to say and I wanted to share all I had discovered. If for no other reason, to let others know some simple things they need to know. Things I wish I'd have known but had to learn the hard way, through the efforts of research and the pain of experience.

I felt if I didn't share this, what about those who couldn't do what I did? What I am doing here? I ran into a few other people with Long Covid who surprised me in just how little info they had, even then. And how badly they wanted to know more.

> Disclaimer: In using an online, Long Covid social media group, I learned to be very careful about what one says, or claims about Long Covid (LC). Even more so than what I felt was normal. The admins there are very careful about what they allowed inside. Covid-19 and long CoVid made me stupid for a while from "brain fog", and exhaustion. Some from fighting it, some from lack of oxygen, all making it hard to think and make decisions. Especially, quick ones.

> We know others have experienced this. Some may even be going through that while reading this book. There is much I will not address in this book, as in many doctor prescribed medicines and other forms Long Covid can take. But, I didn't use those other medicines, and I didn't have those other forms. However, do be aware they are out there. Just because I didn't cover them, doesn't meant they aren't of concern, or relevant to others.

I'll say this for now and I'll say it again later... this is a book on my own personal experiences. On things I discovered that worked for me. So before trying any of this on yourself, it should be presented first to your own doctor. I'll make this too, clear again later on. As with regarding vitamin supplements, which can be very dangerous. This is not a book on all potential considerations or drugs, but on things I have personally experienced and uncovered. This is my story. And if you get nothing else out of it, you will get a way of addressing issues, of how to think about it, to see what's relevant and what's not.

As to who I am...I've been a professional writer, a senior technical writer, an author, a computer/internet/information/software engineer, and a filmmaker. I've written and produced writings and films in documentary, horror and science fiction genres. Covid-19 has been nothing if not a real life horror.

I'm also including some of my history which I've dribbled out over a few books. Enough at first so you know whether I'm worth trusting in this book, and then more than you want or need to know. Maybe I'll gather it all together one day and write my autobio. Not to worry, I'll let you know where I go into that and if you're simply and reasonably just wanting to get into the book's subject, you can skip it.

I've had LC (Long Covid) off and on now, since I first contracted COVID-19 early in February of 2020. After two years of research (out of fear, frustration, painful symptoms and overall irritation and consternation), it occurred to me that I should share what I had found. So I wrote this book in the hope that it may save others some time and effort, and offer in any ways whatsoever, some relief to them, in any way, shape or form. For all those who read it and all those who need it.

More disclaimer...

I'm sharing my findings here to offer things to consider in speaking to your doctor about. Doctors who should be helping with your Long Covid issues. Too many healthcare providers initially ignored LC sufferers to the point of their having died. As we have all learned and become more aware and knowledgeable of it, those numbers have thankfully decreased. Though some haven't. Too many sufferers of LC still cannot find the help they need.

Regarding continuing what seems too difficult (or impossible), my own orientation in life has been that one simply has to do it. As with starting to exercise, again. Especially, after being sedentary for a long period of time. One just has to do it. Just, start. Start brief, build slowly back into it. Then, work to sustain it. And understand that you won't, certainly not at first anyway, be able to exercise as you used to. Perhaps never again. (see, ref# 1 in the reference section)

How? I realized at some point my best chance at curbing this disease, of getting back into shape, was by walking. Once I started, I could get in only a few minutes that first day. I knew if I overdid it, my blood pressure or pulse rate would skyrocket. And that, was pretty scary.

I've had some experiences in my life doing things that felt impossible. College was like that at first, certainly in the consideration of attending higher education. I had graduated high school swearing I'd never go back to school again. But that was mostly because of ADHD when I was younger, Something I hadn't realize until many years later.

Also because K-12 was unduly (and unnecessarily) difficult for me. Honestly though, that was only until about tenth grade when things got easier. I guess by then I had just figured it out. Or my brain (and mind?) had matured/developed enough.

After my years in the USAF, I just figured if I could get through that, I could get through just about anything. It was actually my older brother who talked me into going to college. So once again I signed up for a major life change. One I knew this time would be more relaxed, less dangerous, and yet potentially, far more difficult.

To be sure, at first I found college intimidating. But one just has to take a breath or two and continue. Wisely, I took a study skills class that very first quarter. A wise move indeed. That should be required for every student. And long before college. From there I just had to make getting through each class, each quarter, each year... my one and only goal in life. "Do or die". That, over any or all other things. Like parties. One way or another, I would achieve a college degree regardless anything else.

Without that orientation I could easily and repeatedly have gotten off track. Or when things got tough, just given up. Everything else would have to take a backseat to graduating, to achieving that degree. Everything. Anyone. I found I'd have to apply that thinking to smaller and smaller things. Degree, school years, quarters, classes, research, tests, papers, friends, etc.

My attitude became that I would either graduate, or die: "Graduate or die!" Literally. Sounds foolish now, But once I took that orientation toward college, or any major effort in my life, success became normalized. Looking at it as I did, using the old Samurai mindset of being "all in" (that, "I'm already dead as the battle begins, so fear becomes unnecessary"), I eventually got my two year Associate of Arts degree. Then my university degree.

"Well?" I had thought, "If I could get a two year degree, maybe I could after all achieve a university degree!" I really hadn't planned on a second degree. However, I hadn't really planned on a first degree. My philosophy professor one day told his class that should we choose to go on a university, the work load would be unbelievable.

After making his point, he watched us shrivel in our seats. Only then he added: "But I do believe when called to task, you will all rise to the occasion. You will learn to handle the intensity of studies and manage the workload." We all relaxed. So, I eventually achieved my university degree, too. Honestly, there was a girl involved. Which helped. As that tends to do. But to be fair, we helped one another get through it all (long story, that). I'm not quite sure either of us could have made it alone. For very different reasons.

Thus, regarding my Long Covid exercising, I was sure I could make mere "walking" an acceptable priority to better my health. Walking every day, or every other day as it turned out, as I quickly learned I needed a day between to heal. And my life really did depend on it. To end my LC, or at very least to curb it's misery. LC is so freaking miserable that it really made that effort all the easier. And not exercising enough? That took me back to feeling horrible again. So? There was the motivation.

I mention all this because after so much time being sedentary, floating in a kind of uncomfortable COVID fugue state, it became much easier to fall into the continuing trap of just lying around rather than moving. Or exercising. Or sleeping, which was preferable to being awake and feeling miserable. Although to want to exercise seemed initially to me anyway, as rather counter-intuitive.

Had I not studied toward my degree in college, I wouldn't have felt like I was dying. In order to maintain the thought that dying was my only other option, when you have a disease where so many had actually died, that was just all the more motivating to merely "walk" the other direction, away from the pain (or death). To walk away from the disease. One could say that it's a method of tricking oneself into doing what one wants to do. Though it's really of no matter, as long as you end up doing what you want to do. What you need to do.

With that, I wish you all well!

As I wish us all. And so much so very much more. Because after having a disease such as this (or now, as I still have LC, which is thankfully fading), we all certainly deserve our wellness! Or I should say, no one deserves Long Covid! Well? Either way.

Health! Cheers! Na zdravie! Sláinte!

JZ Murdock

Introduction

COVID-19, as we should all know by now, stands for "Coronavirus Disease 2019". As it was discovered and named in 2019. For ease of use it's typically, "COVID", Covid, or just "covid". You can find various capitalizations in the literature.

> "Coronaviruses are a family of viruses that can cause illnesses such as the common cold, severe acute respiratory syndrome (SARS) and Middle East respiratory syndrome (MERS). In 2019, a new coronavirus was identified as the cause of a disease outbreak that originated in China." Mayo Clinic (see, ref# 2)

Those who have continuing symptoms after COVID-19 has run its course, are referred to as having, "Long Covid". Or, "long haulers disease". Or in the medical literature as: "post-acute sequelae of SARS-CoV-2 infection" or "PASC." What a mouthful.

That initial bout of COVID-19 can be either horrible, deadly, or show no symptoms at all. Some new research is pointing to a relationship with low cortisol levels for those contracting LC. Research is ongoing.

Regardless the duration of LC, aside from its symptomologies, it really becomes another monster all its own. While some have indicated LC can last a couple of years, others seem to get over it much sooner.

It's yet to be seen if some may never be rid of it. Although my own first experience with LC lasted just over a year. Between eight to fourteen months, as it was hard to tell if it was LC or reinfections. I assume now it was just fading LC that would flare up, re-cycling, with ever longer durations between.

Then I caught COVID (and LC again), end of March 2022. And the symptoms were far, far worse, and life threatening.

Key Points of COVID-19

From the CDC:

> • People who are infected but asymptomatic or people with mild COVID-19 should isolate through at least day 5 (day 0 is the day symptoms appeared or the date the specimen was collected for the positive test for people who are asymptomatic). They should wear a mask through day 10. A test-based strategy may be used to remove a mask sooner.

> • People with moderate or severe COVID-19 should isolate through at least day 10. Those with severe COVID-19 may remain infectious beyond 10 days and may need to extend isolation for up to 20 days.

> • People who are moderately or severely immunocompromised should isolate through at least day 20. Use of serial testing and consultation with an infectious disease specialist is recommended in these patients prior to ending isolation. (see, ref# 3)

This book has three main parts. The first, is in these chapters. The last part is an interesting list of reference links. Some are referenced in these chapters, while many others are there for your own reference. In the second half I have include my personal logged daily experiences, from having lived through my own version of Long Covid (or "LC").

What can one get out of reading my daily logs? First, my mental and emotional state. How I was processing all this through those ups and downs as I reacted to those experiences and as I tried new things, or eliminated them.

The logs contain actual and raw data of what happened. What worked and what failed. Sometimes badly and were quite uncomfortable or painful. And there were some surprising results. One that even changed my doctor's mind.

Keeping accurate logs can be very helpful in dealing with our healthcare providers and I highly recommend it. Sadly though, they are not always as helpful with our healthcare provider community as they should, or could be.

Still, more is always better. If and whenever possible.

The four biggest things that helped me with LC?

1. Sleep. Which is odd as in its early stages, I felt I was asleep even when awake and all I seemed to do was sleep.

2. Exercise. Starting as soon as I was able. That took a while, and I needed it sooner than I could do it. To do as much as I could carefully and reasonably do. Then increasing that as I could.

3. Diet. Starting with almost nothing, then adding what seemed reasonable and did not poorly affect me.

4. Finally, medicine ("meds") & vitamin supplements. Which were either life savers, or at times felt like they nearly killed me. Be careful. Don't treat supplements like they're harmless. Or useless.

Some may wish to skip the bulk of this book, jumping ahead just to see the meds or vitamin supplements I used, then move on. To see just what helped me most, or least. That's fine. It's even understandable. As long as it's understood that I'm detailing throughout this book what had helped, ME, in MY situation, with MY symptoms. So if that's not you, you're taking an uncalculated risk in skipping related information.

MY own past physical health history may also be vastly different from yours. Although these things may be of benefit to you, maybe even more so they may not be at all helpful to you. Or even detrimental. And that's in the bulk of this book which will hopefully help to make that all clear to you.

So, ignore all that at your own peril.

As I was writing this book, I came across a new medical white paper (net yet peer reviewed at the time I read it). It was about people who were shown to acquire Long Covid with low levels of cortisol.

Extrapolating from that and in looking cortisol up, I found zinc and pantothenic acid supplements (and a couple other things), that might help with Long Covid. This kind of speculation can be helpful, or beyond useless, to dangerous. So from here one must move forward carefully. But that's also how one can find things that do help. Careful, informed speculation, reviewing perhaps with your doctor, and testing it out. For you.

Unproven, not yet peer reviewed, not yet replicated. However at this point, with still so little knowledge about LC, when you're suffering through it you do tend to experiment on yourself. As I did. I wish I had known about this before however. Or two years ago. I did try taking zinc in the beginning, when I first contracted LC. But it didn't seem to help. Though perhaps I should have kept it up?

You shouldn't use zinc long term, however. I tried the zinc recently after reading about it, but the effect wasn't very pleasant. So I stopped. The trouble with LC is that at times when something does work, it can feel for a bit like it's going the other direction. Just as with starting to exercise. One can even feel ill for a bit, or sore for a few days. But you have to keep it up. Push through it. Carefully, if you can. While many just give up. However, be also extremely aware that at times "pushing through" LC, can be dangerous. It's yet another thing that makes this disease so insidious.

In my daily logs, a few times I described eating "normally". Or perhaps saying I "ate too much" of something over the length of a day. The reason for that was two fold.

First, to check my progress on how healthy I was at the time. But also to "feed" my intense desire to feel normal again (both in my actions and habits). Perhaps incorrectly. But that desire after two years had become strong in my being sick to death of not being able to be and act normal. It's hard to explain that feeling. But not to someone who has LC, for any length of time.

Some of those experiences, I shared, emailing them to my Veterans Administration doctor. Though I don't think he appreciated it too much. Since when he finally responded back he mentioned how they're not a research facility. Well, point taken I guess. Though I wish that weren't the case. Patients, especially knowledgeable ones, can be a great benefit to healthcare professionals.

However, some of us (too many?) can indeed be counter productive, jamming up healthcare for others. I'm sure doctors and nurses regularly deal with that to a rather disconcerting degree. They may very well reasonably assume you or I are simply yet another who will waste their time, delaying them getting to their next appointment. Medical professionals who hear, "I searched the internet", or perhaps worse, "I researched it myself on the internet", just has to strike fear in the heart of many a nurse or doctor. And again, reasonably so.

As I'm not a doctor, I'm making my own best guesses about all of this. Just as everyone else does. Including as I've discovered, some medical researchers and professionals. While I'm not claiming to be one of those, my background does give me a little more credibility than most citizen researchers.

I can be very focused and I have a generally more informed consideration and outlook of research and information I find than most do. My conclusions are considered and then reconsidered, and when possible (when information/references are available), cross-referenced. I try to find problematic issues with them. I also try to keep an opened and focused mind.

I will lay out here what I've gone through and comment as best I can on what seems most logical and reasonable. Backed up by research and the medical profession wherever possible. I'll show most of my work, including findings in comments and weblinks. Some referencing hard science "white papers". But I've tried to keep that to a minimum, for the sake of most. Or summarize what I've found.

To some, my daily logs will be of great use. To most? Well, maybe not so much. Or at all. I do know they would be of great use to me if I had come across them, from someone else. But that's me and I have a degree in psychology.

So I include these logs here in my due diligence to include all relevant material available to me. They are at times interesting, insightful, pedantic and humorous and I include them for the sake of posterity and in the event they may offer even one person a little insight. One never knows what will.

If nothing else, one can see how someone else had gone through this and is going through it. It may make you feel better in some way or another.

Reading a social media LC support group evoked some comfort for me. But as well compassion for they who were having a much worse go of it. Hopefully things I said in that group helped some there to feel better.

They also put my own suffering in perspective. In lessening its perceived intensity in my own info vacuum, regarding their living anecdotes. To be honest, perhaps allowing me a healthy degree of apathy in accepting where I was at rather than always comparing it to where I wanted to be. Which can just make one miserable. Mostly though it helped me to hear other's experiences and know I was not alone. COVID and LC, along with social isolation, has left many to feel all too singular and separated.

These logs are at times merely data and mundane, especially in the beginning. Other times they border on journaling, or a diary. They definitely detail the misery I went through, the fears I had, and the hope I tried to keep alive. This was the longest period of time I've ever experienced with concerns over whether I would be alive the next day, or the next hour. Or not.

I have read there are over 200 symptoms that can be combined to be called, "Long Covid", which can be triggered by COVID-19. As I see it, if I can catch COVID, I can get over it (not yet so true, but it does help one to keep striving). As one begins to heal from a COVID infection, it can take a virus that has long lain dormant within your system from previous infections, and activate it.

 Possibly even a virus from childhood, or birth, triggering it back into action. It is in part whey the medical profession has been misled and confused over COVID so often. It's not medical incompetence, but COVID complexity.

That triggering may evoke something like Epstein-Barr (EBV). Or something else which causes the symptoms. Epstein-Barr is, according to the CDC: "...also known as human herpes virus 4, a member of the herpes virus family. It is one of the most common human viruses."

> From NIH: "According to epidemiological studies, the EBV is estimated to be positive in more than 90% of the world's populations (4). Typically, the primary infection is asymptomatic and occurs during childhood." NIH are the

National Library of Medicine, National Center for Biotechnology Information.

From there, one reasonably wants to alleviate the symptoms which can be infuriatingly uncomfortable. If you can reduce or eliminate those symptoms, you still have to get rid of, deactivate, the triggered virus(es).

Solving how to deactivate a triggered virus is not the same as ending COVID-19. Symptoms can be mixed, can come and go. Long Covid itself can recycle through, coming and going for weeks, months, or years on end. Potentially for some, remaining with them for good. We're still in the early history of LC eventualities. Thinking you're finally over it, then it recycles back on you, can feel devastating.

Long Covid is a frustrating condition that's difficult to pin down. It can have any combination of a variety of symptoms. Once you think you're over it, it may return in days, weeks, or months. Hopefully not, years later. As it's only been in our consciousness for a few of years at this time, we still have much to learn about it in the longer term. If these last two paragraphs seem redundant, well...welcome to LC.

Obviously, I didn't keep a log when COVID first hit me. I was too sick. Too exhausted all the time. Which I now know was from suffering low oxygen levels, as well as being tired from my immune system being constantly in overdrive fighting something at times it wouldn't recognize as disease.

Until my immune system itself may have started attacking me. COVID can trick your immune system. Which was why mine didn't even know to have a fever to help fight it off. Or why it felt like the inside surfaces of my veins were being attacked, like acid were surging through them.

I will briefly go over how I first acquired it and how over the next two years, I suffered through LC. Then infuriatingly I caught COVID at least once more (maybe twice?). Maybe more than that, as my immunity or vaccines may have fought off other infection(s) when acquired, or acquired with viral loads small enough to defeat it. It's really hard to determine, if not impossible.

Long Covid seemed to last a long time that first year of 2020, and into the next. It would come and travel in waves, or cycles. I'd have it for a week, or three, then have a week off, or three. Then back again. So every month I was experiencing Long Covid for one to three (plus) weeks. It was frustrating. Disparaging. I was so lethargic that the year passed much faster than I would ever have guessed.

I was born on a warm, cloud covered and somewhat drizzly Tuesday, on August 30th of 1955. As of this writing, I'm 67 years old. Which had something to do with my (in)ability to initially fight off COVID, as well as in catching LC.

On the other hand, I had somehow avoided a cytokine storm (or receiving bad enough damages from it), fighting the disease off well enough that I survived. Apparently without serious life long repercussions (though it may be yet to be seen years, or decades from now).

> Cytokine storm and cytokine release syndrome are life-threatening systemic inflammatory syndromes involving elevated levels of circulating cytokines and immune-cell hyperactivation that can be triggered by various therapies, pathogens, cancers, autoimmune conditions, and monogenic disorders. (see, ref# 4)

I positively caught COVID again, on about Sunday, March 28, 2022. I couldn't tell after my first infection if other possible infections were actually new infections, or simply Long Covid, recyclese. If you like closure in life, COVID really isn't for you.

I ended up calling paramedics for the first time in my life, at 2AM that next morning. I found later I had been experiencing, "sinus tachycardia" (normal rhythm, with heartbeats over 100 beats per minute). It was over 160BPM, for no apparent reason (to me). After the paramedics left, with my VA Nurse's suggestion, I eventually headed to the nearest Emergency Department, at a hospital in the next town over. More on that nightmare (and getting there), later.

A week later, I had to call paramedics again, and again it was 2AM. This time for blood pressure being too high. It got up to 168/88. Looking it up online in that moment, I found two reliable references saying if/when it got to 160, call 911.

Within twenty minutes, it went back up to that so I called 911. But by time they arrived, it had gone back down to the high end of normal. Both times, had I just waited, I wouldn't have had to call 911. But that's the miserable thing. If you don't call and it doesn't go back down, you could die. Something at the time that felt all too possible sitting at home, alone, in the middle of the night.

To be accurate regarding blood pressure (FDA.gov):

> "Normal pressure is 120/80 or lower. Your blood pressure is considered high (stage 1) if it reads 130/80. Stage 2 high blood pressure is 140/90 or higher. If you get a blood pressure reading of 180/110 or higher more than once, seek medical treatment right away."

So, maybe I could have waited. Which exemplifies two things. Whenever you need to know something in an emergency (or a perceived emergency), it's best to know those things ahead of time. And be careful what you find online. To be fair, I was a little shaken. It was two o'clock in the morning. I was tired and not thinking straight. Plus, the condition and it's history both added to my physical and emotional state, and mental stress and confusion.

After paramedics left that second time, I called the Veterans Association Healthcare triage Nurse. I spoke with her at length and she decided this time I was probably, OK. I did not need to go to the ED again. But if it rose like that again, she said I should call 911, again. And that time she said, go with the ambulance to the ED and get checked out. Obviously, the first time I called paramedics, the VA Nurse said I should go to the hospital, which I did.

So it was at that point when I started digging deeper into Long Covid research going forward. Beyond what I had already done over the past two years. What the hell was going on? For the next weeks and months my VA doctor had me go in for various lab tests. All came back looking unexpectedly normal. Apparently, I was healthy. Still. Yet, somehow I wasn't. Obviously, I was at a loss, and so was he.

There were no VA Long Covid teams (not in Washington, anyway) to handle people going through what I was. I found that unbelievable! To be fair, it's a small percentage of us who contract LC. But one doesn't much care when you're suffering through it.

Again from the CDC:

> "Overall, 1 in 13 adults in the U.S. (7.5%) have "Long Covid" symptoms, defined as symptoms lasting three or more months after first contracting the virus, and that they didn't have prior to their COVID-19 infection. Older adults are less likely to have long COVID than younger adults. Jun 22, 2022"

That, was disappointing. So, I'm in an even smaller cohort at my age, having LC. Great. Still, that all left me with whatever tools I had at my disposal, and an ability to do my own research. It was just a matter of finding the energy and wherewithal to do the boring (and at times, disturbing) research. One does have to be careful not to see the worst in your symptoms and go off the deep end. As many do with online research. It's become rather a cliché since the advent of the internet.

In 2016 I retired from a frontline IT engineer team (information/ internet technologies) at Regence BlueShield. A four state (Washington, Oregon, Idaho, Utah) health insurance company regarded as a "Cadillac of health insurance". I had been in IT for decades as a tech writer, a senior programmer/analyst, various types of software/network administrators, and as a software/ platform engineer.

However, my Western Washington University degree is in psychology, in their department's Awareness and Reasoning division, concentrating in phenomenology. Leading me one time to joke to my IT team, when asked how (why?) I went from psychology to computers.

They all had computer science or math degrees. But I told them that troubleshooting a computer was a lot like doing the same with people. They stared at me for a moment, then laughed. You could see them one by one, seeing the relevance. I was actually very good at troubleshooting and fixing things. More than once I helped one of our programmers find a fault in their programming when they were stumped, and I didn't even know that programming language.

My university degree offers me a good background both for clinical observation, as well as research. Even to some degree in medical issues, and to observations of myself. As that is much of what phenomenology is. Or certainly can be in observing one's human experience.

> "A whole family of qualitative methods is informed by phenomenological philosophy. When applying these

methods, the material is analyzed using concepts from this philosophy to interrogate the findings and to enable greater theoretical analysis. However, the phenomenological approach represents different approaches, from pure description to those more informed by interpretation." - NIH, Phenomenological Approaches in Psychology and Health Sciences (see, ref# 5)

It's the observation of interactions of humans to phenomena throughout their existence in the world, and out of it. A fascinating area for research and study. My seminal university paper in my senior level abnormal psychology seminar (a small senior level class) was studying schizophrenia through synesthesia, and vice versa (see my ebook, "On Psychology: With Illustration in Psychopathology via Synesthesia and Schizophrenia", available on Smashwords and Amazon, link under my personal links in the last section of this book).

All of my efforts as detailed in this book may well have lessened, certainly the intensity of my symptoms, but also potentially the duration of my LC. That may very well be as true as not as it's a hard thing to prove in either direction.

What I do know is I have indeed lessened the severity of my symptoms, so far seemingly for its duration. No matter how long that lasts. Yes, I did get the updated booster that finally came out September of 2022. Possibly, I will even get another in the future. Or from now on, just as we now have annual flu shots. Unless newer discoveries become available, negating our need for COVID vaccines. (see, ref# 6)

Introduction

Chapter 1

My Background

What follows in this section is not for purposes of ego, but to exemplify my contentions that I have some qualitative background as a mere citizen, so that I can reasonably be considered in my contentions here, regarding medical and experiential issues. That is to say, one can have some degree of trust in what I'm saying in this book.

Also, some may see themselves (or others they know) in what I describing here and may (hopefully) gain some understanding and insight.

I was a very active kid. Too active. An overly active ADHD kid. In asking my mother once why she always had me as a kid, taking one kind of after school lesson or another, she told me she had quickly learned she needed to wear me down every day. Just so I'd go to sleep at night.

One might also assume that getting me out of the house (and her immediate environment), was healthy for us both. Just in giving her a break from me if nothing else. Something I learned with my own son who she once told me was like watching a little me running around.

She also liked to say that if she put me down to sleep at 5AM, I'd be back up at 6AM. My own son was much the same.

The main point I'm sharing in this section is that I have ADHD and was very active as a kid (obviously). I had a physically active first part of my life. Martial arts, backpacking, search and rescue, and beginning my work life at fourteen when alone, I daily cleaned up the field of a drive-in theater for a season. Ever day of

the week. Back breaking work.

Which research has shown, a lot of physicality in our younger child and adult years lends itself to better health in our later years. An active mind can also be good for fighting off the affects of aging on the brain. Which actively guided my life and career choices toward having as functional a mind as possible in my old age. That is, I exercised a lot in life and chose difficult mentally challenging jobs, with the thought of growing old one day.

At this point, please do feel free to skip this entire section which is just more nonsense about myself.

Unless you're simply curious about my background or need further assurance on my...bone fides, my credentials, I think most have gotten the main points by now that I was trying to make.

The following are just more specific historical and personal information.

As a kid, I had trouble sleeping ("...down at 5AM, up at 6AM."). My mind always seemed to be racing and kept me awake at night. I got bored talking to people because I was always a couple of sentences/concepts ahead of them and had to wait for them to catch up. Which meant at times I'd get lost waiting for them, which oddly could make me appear stupid to some. Like my step-father.

To those who recognized that, I did get more attention and care. That is, they would pick up the pace. I really only remember three teachers in high school who recognized that. To this day I have fond affection for them. I only remember one grade school teacher, in sixth grade, who saw that, saw something, and was of great help toward my being more successful in junior high and especially in high school.

Sleepwise, the worst was in my high school years. I'd lie in bed wishing for sleep, watching hours slip by until my alarm went off. Typically allowing me only a few frustrating hours of sleep. Too often sleep was merely dozing all night. Of course I did get some good nights of sleep, here and there. But as I worked nights at the drive-in theater all through high school, there was no time to "wind down" before hoping into bed and hoping for sleep.

So by time I got into bed, my mind would still be racing from work. I remember lying in bed imagining ways to knock myself out. Suffocation? No. I also didn't want to die. The only answer was getting enough exercise during the day. Which at times, ironically left me too tired to fall asleep, anyway. It's a weird thing when you are thoroughly exhausted, but too exhausted to fall asleep.

What can lead to that kind of insomnia? Stress and anxiety (probably, I was a teenager), over stimulation (definitely, snack bar work at a drive-in theater is nothing if not that), sleep disorders (ADHD), circadian rhythm disruption (working nights), physical discomfort or pain (sometimes from being on my feet, running around waiting on people), medication or stimulants (I didn't have that issue.

ADHD sleep symptoms: Hyperarousal, Racing Thoughts, Delayed Sleep Phase, Restlessness, Coexisting Conditions. Good times...which all made for a need to fight not to fall asleep in class. I actually discovered one day in twelfth grade that I could fall asleep in class, chin on hand holding me up, sleeping with my eyes open and my teacher never noticed. Also, when you are sleep deprived you slip into "micro-naps" (or, "microsleeps"). Dangerous during periods of driving a car.

My dreams were many and varied, ever since I was young. I found them quite entertaining. I read a lot of science fiction as a kid, no doubt enhancing those dreams. While awake, my imagination was typically overactive. Too active, as befits an ADHD kid in being often bored in class, staring out windows, not paying attention, mostly a problem in elementary school.

I remember once in sixth grade telling my older sister that I couldn't wait to go to sleep that night, to see where my dreams would take me. They were just so interesting, fascinating. Her comment was, "That's really sad. Your life is so boring you can't wait to go to sleep? Really?" She looked genuinely sad for me. She was always a great example of a big sister.

Bored? I hadn't considered that I found my life boring, or seen it in that way. Replying to her I said, "Well, maybe. But you don't know how cool my dreams are!" Which just got me a sideways glance from her as she walked away, unsure what it was I was going through.

Being half-siblings in having different dads, we were similar but quite different (each of my siblings). But then, female ADHD kids can present quite differently than boys. She was the straight "A" student, obviously attractive with a far different school life growing up than I had. My guy friends seeing my older sister for the first time, or a photo of her, would look at me and taunt, "Guess we can see who got all the good looks between you two."

I was taunted a lot as a kid. I asked a guy once about that in high school and he was honest with me about it. He said he liked me and liked teasing me because my reactions were so fun. In being smaller than the other kids until about 10th grade when I shot up to 6' (eventually 6'2"), I had been bulled a bit and learned to use humor. My older brother once told me that self-deprecating humor was a good way to get out of sticky situations. Knock yourself down before a bully has the chance to. And he was right. So I became a kind of entertainer. Also, our mother had a great sense of humor.

About my siblings, all of us who had different fathers, while we were all massively beloved siblings between us and with our mother. My sister seemed to always do the right things. She gave the best presents in the world. People seeing our looks would tease how she must have gotten all the looks in our family. When I followed her into high school (I entered the year after she left), teachers were shocked or surprised I was related to her.

Our older brother seven years my senior wasn't often with us, being raised mostly by his authoritarian father. Our youngest brother five years my junior, died of liver cancer only two weeks from his fifteenth birthday, in a Manhattan hospital, in July 1975. Months later in September, I entered USAF basic training as a "Vietnam era" enlistee with those full benefits where I eventually received the rank of Staff Sergeant and a Good Conduct medal.

For myself, I leaned more toward being the problem kid. A good kid, a happy kid, and a generally well liked one, but always with a little something off. Or as my sister frequently and somewhat affectionately would put it, "You're so weird."

That confused me because I heard it a lot from various people growing up. Whenever I heard that I would reflect where I heard or read what I had just said, if I were referring to something or someone else which they were responding to. Frequently it was from some great thinker I had read.

Like Aristotle, who I got into in fifth grade at the library. Or Isaac Asimov, Or other sci fi writers now considered our greatest golden age science fiction writers. Or relating some pure science, as I was very into NASA and the space program in the 1960s. If only that had all properly translated into my school work, and my grades.

It wasn't until 10th grade when I discovered I wasn't actually stupid, or "slow". Though not quite, "retarded" (pretty typical wor back then), as no one really thought that (except my step-father). As it turned out, my classroom was simply too slow for me to follow. Which was counter-intuitive.

I finally realized that one day in my tenth grade English

Composition class. We were getting a complicated lesson from our teacher who was zipping along at the blackboard. I suspect, she was just enjoying herself, losing herself in writing out her instruction.

Suddenly, I had perked up. I felt energized. I leaned forward, feeling highly engaged. But suddenly, the entire class as one loudly exclaimed that they were lost. To please slow down. That startled me, sitting in the front row.

This was the same great teacher who, at the beginning of the year, told us "if you have trouble following along in class, don't hide in back. Sit up front where there's less distractions". I thought that made sense. So I moved forward which was indeed a great help. Ignoring my social discomfort, but becoming better able to pay attention during class time.

The class complained that she had been too fast and several asked aloud for her to slow down. I was despondent and actually exclaimed out loud myself, as if hurt, "Please, don't slow down! I was just getting it!"

But reasonably the majority shouted me down and won out. Still, it was from that day on that I finally realized what had been going on all my life. Why my classes were so often so difficult for me. It wasn't boredom, per se. It wasn't low IQ. Instruction was just so often too painfully slow for me that I'd lose track by time the teacher got to their point. So in a way, it was boring for me.

To perhaps further clarify this, in 8th grade I, along with my classmates, lucked into being taught in an Evelyn Wood Reading Dynamics experiment where they taught us their techniques in a classroom environment. I had switched from public school to a private Catholic parochial school. Eighth grade being the final grade there. So we were taught their method over one school quarter.

We were tested that first on our reading comprehension, then again at the end. I went from 250 words per minute with 60% comprehension, to 10,000 words per minute and 80% comprehension. Eventually, I stopped using it by the end of my next year in 9th grade.

Why? Because I honestly got tired of reading a novel within an hour, or less. It was cool. though. It was like watching a movie in your head, very different from normal reading. Especially when you hear the words you read in your head, slowing down your reading speed. They had taught us that's the first thing you have to stop doing because one does not need to "hear" the words in one's head, in order to understand the words.

I came to realize I preferred to take my time to assimilate a story, a book a novel. I enjoyed considering the story during and between chapters. For a week, if possible. Or at least for a few days. I wanted time to consider it, relish it, reflect on certain passages a few times before going to the next section. The more beloved the book, the longer I wanted the book to last before moving onto a new book.

Later on, at twenty-one, and while in the USAF, I took the class again. I saw they were teaching a class downtown Spokane, Washington which I was based near. I lived downtown with my wife. After graduating that first class in eighth grade, they gave us all a letter. I still have it. It says that we could take their class again, any time we wished, and for the rest of our lives. For free.

So I took it again, just for fun. Because even knowing I had done it before, having lived through doing it, knowing it was real, I still found it hard to believe those many years later that I had actually been able to read that fast. But I had. We did. And then, I did it again. The teacher that first day in Spokane at the beautiful, historic Davenport hotel introduced me to the class of about thirty people. He told them I was proof the course works. I answered some questions, and then we got down to it.

That need for speed, all worked out very well for me later in life. Both in IT, as a technical writer, as a fiction writer, and now even as a filmmaker.

Regarding physical exercise as a kid. I started Isshinryu Karate from the very famous martial artist, Steve Armstrong, beginning in 5th grade. I became a "dojo rat", being there as much as I could be. A requirement at the dojo was to compete in tournaments around the Pacific Northwest to support our dojo (school).

When we first heard that at the dojo we were all terrified. But it all turned into an ongoing, rewarding experience. In college in the early 80s, I switched martial arts from Okinawan Karate to Japanese Aikido, when introduced to it for the first time in a physical education elective.

I'd never heard of Aikido before, but it's the one true Japanese martial art (Judo, being a sport). Eventually, I found a local Kitsap County dojo when I moved over here in 2000. Eventually I joined their board of directors when one was created for our 501(c)(3), non- profit school.

I studied Karate as a kid for several years, competing in many tournaments around the Pacific Northwest. Until my attention turned to something more aerospace oriented.

In 8th grade I learned about and immediately joined the Civil Air Patrol, an auxiliary of the USAF. We met monthly. At the second meeting I was given the manual and told there was a lot of new cadets suddenty and they needed another Flight Commander for our new second flight, and I was he. I had one month to learn the entire manual and then teach it to the other only slightly newer cadets. Terrified, in the end I succeeded.

We wore kid-sized, full official USAF uniforms. During WWII, the C.A.P. was founded when civilian pilots flew our coasts checking for enemy vessels. Over the years it had evolved into much more. It gave a great foundation for many kids who saved a lot of lives, or recovered those in lost, downed small aircraft.

At first I play acted my role as Flight Commander, but I quickly fell into doing a rather good job of it and become more self-assured. Something I really needed. I was also very happy about my previous dojo experiences as I had trained a lot of the new kids.

Eventually, I became our Tacoma, Washington squadron's 1st Sergeant. I learned to sign up for any available training I could get, in all elements of aerospace technologies and organized search and rescue. We trained in our "local" Cascade Mountains. I was also able to train with our elite statewide "Wing Team". We would receive training a week at at time, at their base in the Olympic Mountains. Not far from where I live today.

Later, in US Air Force basic training, my time in CAP landed me a position as squad leader. The most important one, right front position in a marching formation (also as I was tallest in a standard "flight" of fifty basic trainees, or "Airmen Basic"), as everyone takes their tempo off of you. More or less.

It was sad however, when I ws told that I would not receive my first stripe in rank, while in basic training. It seems I was only a month short of my time in CAP for that. Had I only known that as a kid, I would have kept that option open and remained a bit longer. Our CAP squadron had been falling apart when too many of our "Seniors" who were active military had been transferred out to other bases around the world. So I lost interest in the chaos and quit.

When one has been in CAP long enough and rose high enough in rank, a USAF Airman Basic can graduate basic training with up to two stripes. While most graduate as "slick sleeves" with no stripes, one can receive one stripe to "Airman", or two stripes for

"Airman First Class". Three stripes, which used to be called "Sergeant", is now known as Senior Airman and takes putting in time served later on at one's main base of station.

I was in CAP in 1968 when I took pilot/flight "ground school" (twice actually, they had to cancel the first training half way through, for some reason) and I got to fly in and pilot small aircraft myself around the PNW. I even got to land the plane once at Tacoma Industrial Airport (now, Tacoma Narrows Airport), near the Tacoma Narrows Bridge.

Landing at TNA was an amazing experience, especially for a kid. Especially that day as my cadet First Sergeant had a cast on his broken leg. He had to sit uncomfortably in the back seat, and was terrified for me to land the plane. But our pilot, an active duty USAF officer, assured him it would be fine. And it was.

We spent time in CAP bivouacking/backpacking in the mountains, learning first responder first aid and practicing search and rescue techniques. These included the basics of "LSAR" (Land Search and Rescue), "Communications" (between command and those on the ground searching, and search aircraft above), as well as "Ground Support" of aircraft, used to survey for lost/downed aircraft.

Backpacking was integral and a pastime that followed me into adulthood. I also earned my "Radio Telegraph Operators" license for operating HAM radio around the world. Typically, we used CB radios in the field, which I also became proficient in. This was long before their popularity they received later in the 1970s by way of popular Hollywood films.

I started working the summer before 9th grade, at thirteen, at the drive-in theater our step-father worked at after his day job. First, I would pick up the field trash each day before the next showing that evening. Then later, I was a snack bar worker and finally I rose to snack bar manager and later, box office cashier, replacing my step-father when he moved with the manager to the then new and shiny, 112th Street Drive-in Theater.

Graduating high school at seventeen, I acquired a job at an insurance company (United Pacific Insurance, which later merged with east coast Reliance Insurance to become United Pacific Reliance Insurance). It was also my sister's first, post-high school job. She recently retired as a Sr. Flight Attendant, only her second job. She also worked at the drive-in before me. I then moved out of my parents' house at seventeen, and into my first apartment.

It's notable that I have written a seven time multi-international award winning screenplay that I am currently shopping around. Titled, "The Teenage Bodyguard", it is a true crime/biopic that has received a True Crime Podcast episode ("Scene of the Crime - "The Enterprise") and attention from several directors and a producer. That true story took place at that point in my life within a year of moving out of my parents house.

That next year at eighteen, I started sky diving. I had already become a certified NAUI SCUBA diver back early in 11th grade. This was the second time in my life, oddly enough, where a group came to a school I was attending to experiment in teaching in an educational setting rather than at their own facility.

I then took foil fencing that year at the YWCA with my mom, my sister our younger brother. Our mom was so motivated by my getting a SCUBA license, that she and my sister got certified, and then wanted us to do more family activities together. Thus, fencing. Which pretty much sadly, ended that streak. Perhaps in part because our youngest brother had become ill which we later discovered was terminal.

I had also been on our high school rifle team, through all three years of high school and from which I received my high school sports "letter" from (a gold and black "L" for Lincoln High School).

It's funny. I always thought I wasn't doing much of anything back then. But now, looking back? It seems like I kind of did a lot. After working for a while and living on my own, I quit my job and I traveled America a bit. I spent time in Phoenix, Manhattan, Jersey City, Spokane, Denver, Vancouver, British Columbia, Canada, and a few other places.

I tried out as a Tacoma Policeman at nineteen. I took their written test and obstacle course. I didn't get a job. But then I didn't know people actually bought books and studied for the written exam. Though I was first to finish (with a bit of a gap to the next fastest time) on their obstacle course, at times literally flying over parts (or under).

Finally, wanting more direction and options in life, I joined the USAF. I didn't see any possibility in my life of really getting anywhere, as things were. I was twenty and signed up as "guaranteed job", Law Enforcement. Not as "SP" or Security Police who mostly guarded things.

Alas, I was canceled from that job and ended up as a second choice as parachute rigger because of "flat feet". Packing chutes was a physical job. Especially packing 228 pound, B-52 drag chutes which could get rather grueling. Especially, when they were rain soaked, or had scooped up snow in the winter time. Every work day, for that first year or so, usually all morning long, I packed those drag chutes as the newest kid in the shop.

At times I'd have to pack them all day, every day when it was during ORI "alerts" (Operational Readiness Inspections). These tested the functionality of an airbase for activating instantly for war. Then I could pack up to fourteen per day, for an entire week. Obviously, when I separated service I was in the best physical conditioning of my life. While I had to sign a document swearing not to share any secret information I'd had access to with my secret level clearance, twenty-five years have now long passed.

Our job was to get several B-52s and a Stratotanker into the air in the first fifteen minutes, as if we were at war. Then as many more planes in the air before being nuked ourselves by the "enemy". We excelled at our jobs.

Beyond drag chutes, I had other duties. Those included inspecting/packing emergency personnel chutes for high speed deployments, and inspecting/packing parachutes for Pararescue personnel. Those are the famous USAF PJs who fight into a battle to extract the wounded. These are Tough Guys. And the nicest guys I ever knew or worked with. Their chutes I packed were jumped daily, typically from helicopters.

Aside from packing chutes, I worked to maintain and prep uploaded nuclear B-52 bombers and KC-135 Stratotankers, readying them to take flight for war at a moment's notice. I held a Secret clearance for nuclear weapons on the USAF PRP/HRP (for Personal or Human Reliability) programs, for being on and around nuclear weapons. Which could literally get you killed if you stepped over the wrong line on the ground.

Here's a brief aside you'll never hear anywhere else. The year before the end of my USAF term of service in October 1978, I had my initial interviews over a month or so, with the Commanding Officer of our base OSI office toward becoming an OSI Agent. They are the USAF version of the FBI.

I in fact, read "FBI" magazine sitting in their waiting room. I tested extremely well he said, and the CO and I got along. This is a much longer story, but I mention it for one story that happened back then in Europe he shared with me.

When he was trying to find what I was interested in career-wise, and what base location in the world best suited me and that I wanted, we ended up settling on Berlin.

Why? Because, I said I wanted to learn field work. "Berlin, then."

he said, "It's the best place in the world for that. In fact, there's an opening there now, if you're interested. It's been open for over a year now. If you put in for it, you'll probably get it."

"Really?" I realized there was a thread there to pull. "Why has it been open so long? How come no one wants that job?" Berlin was a center for much between the Soviets and western democracies. "Yes," he said, "but it seems the last agent died on the job and no one wants to replace him"

Curious, I pushed further. "How did he die?"

"Car bomb."

"Car bomb? Who would blow up an OSI agent?" He nodded his head slowly and raised an eyebrow. I felt I should know what that meant. And I did. But I pushed him to say it aloud. "Who?" He looked at me somewhat confused.

"You know."

"The KBG? Blew up an agent?" He nodded.

"That's why no one wants the job. Apparently. I mean...it's been a long while now and the position is still vacant. That's pretty unusual." We stared at one another a long moment.

"Well? Sign me up, then."

"Are you sure?"

"Yes, sure. I want to learn [my lifelong mantra]. That looks like the place for it." I still have the document he signed, indicating my assignment choice: Berlin.

Sadly, it wasn't meant to be. My choice due to family issues. But it does make for an interesting story, now.

That was the first half of my life, I lived a fairly physical existence. I was in good health. Minus whatever I may have taken with me from my time in Service, in being around and maintaining weapons of war. Something I knew that later, one day, might take a toll on me. There were plenty of toxic substances and radiation. Did any of that cost me in this current COVID scenario?

My point in mentioning all this? It's been noted in medical literature that those who have had a lot of physical exercise in their formative and early adult years, fare much better in their elder years. My health has been pretty much above normal, all of my life. Even now, through all this. Am I an outlier? Hard to tell.

In that sense, I may be above normal in my health issues. Which is important. As COVID is not easy on those who have not led healthy lives. Or were not above normal in physical conditioning in their younger years. Or those who are currently not in the best of health, or have pre-existing conditions.

Many who are obese or have a dormant or active disease, or are in poor health in general, have died from COVID. Some even from LC, apparently. That's all been noted in the medical literature. But those are for specific group types, which most of us won't need to be overly concerned about. As most of us in general also won't have to worry much about LC, either.

Through these past two years, due to COVID, all the tests I've been given have shown me still to be in the best of health, For my cohort, my age group. There are more tests however being made known to us.

As in using PET scans of inner heart muscle tissue to detect damaged, unrecoverable cells. Research on COVID continues as more avenues for prognosis are discovered and released to medical professionals, and the public. (see ref# 7)

Chapter 1

Chapter 2

COVID-19, A Strangely Novel Infection

As I've mentioned, I first acquired COVID on February 9, 2020, a Sunday. It began with a sinus headache. I have had normal seasonal allergy issues all my life. As many do. But it did seem worse after my USAF years of breathing in JP-4 jet fuel exhaust, off of inspecting and repacking of B-52 bomber drag chutes.

While packing them within a typically closed room, with poor (maybe no?) ventilation. The medical literature has yet to explore that. Or note that it has been an issue with other riggers of B-52 drag chutes. Or other military jet drag chutes of any kind. Which as we've learned the hard way, time and again, doesn't mean they doesn't exist.

Considering we had been told for years that the "Agent Orange" America used in Vietnam was, "harmless", while the military knew different. Until we issues about heavy metals in the spinal cord were made public.

As well as the more recent "gaslighting" regarding burn pits near battlefields were "harmless" in war because they were so easy and useful to the military. How a burn pit filled with items of toxic ingredients of war, could ever have been considered, "safe", is quite beyond one's rational mind.

My initial bout of COVID lasted about five to six days. Then with time, it faded away (that is, I healed) through several stages of onset, peak symptoms, and healing. At some point during all that, Long Covid had set in before I realized it.

COVID had hit in one day, as I said, on a Sunday. By the next day, it had briefly moved into my throat throughout that day and by nighttime it had settled into my chest. But in a way I had never experienced before. And I was familiar with annual bronchitis as

17

a kid. But something about this felt very different. Now it's one of my COVID considerations. If you're sick and it feels different than anything you've ever had before, it may be COVID. Get it checked.

By that Tuesday, it was fully involved in my chest, making sleep very difficult because of the need to breathe without coughing. I learned quickly to avoid that if possible. Monday, Tuesday, and Wednesday nights were horrible experiences. Each night worse than the previous.

I would lie awake in bed, carefully trying to breathe, minute after minute, all night long. It was frustrating. It was exhausting. By the third night of that, I was becoming seriously concerned. Partly because I was so exhausted and knowing that had to be affecting my immune system.

During that week I had been telling friends and family on social media that I did not have the flu. This was something new. Something...disturbing. Mostly I got polite, compassionate comments to try and relax about it and let it pass. What can you say to something like that?

People said it was probably just the flu, or some local respiratory infection that was going around. They didn't know better then, none of us did. We didn't even know it was in Washington state until later when it was announced two had died at Life Care Center in Kirkland, 23 miles from me, on February 26th, fourteen days after I could have, nearly died of it, myself.

Pretty quickly I realized I couldn't convince anyone about what it was. Or how bad it was. I just sounded like a complainer. So I didn't push it and stopped mentioning it. Just every so often I'd say something to point out I still had whatever it was. By that time I was into Long Covid.

Then we started to hear more details about it on the news, about what it was. We all learned more about it together over the next months and year.

Each day more intensely affirmed my conviction that this was indeed some new disease. Probably that disease we were hearing about. It was a stunning discovery. At first there were a few things released, something about China, maybe.

But that was China. Right? So all I could do was lie in my recliner in the living room, watch TV and fool around online on my laptop, intermittently, uncontrollably falling asleep. It took a lot of concentration to do anything substantive. I didn't realize yet that part of the problem was low oxygen levels.

That third and final night of COVID proper, I was lying in bed, exhausted, alone, staring at the bedside clock as the hours ticked by, I began to wonder if I should drive to the emergency department? Should I drive the two miles to the local St. Michael's Medical Center in east Bremerton?

That was the hospital where I had taken my kids over the past couple of decades whenever they needed a hospital. Which wasn't often. Back then we were twenty-three miles from it in Suquamish, where Chief Seattle is buried. So, I knew the hospital well enough. But I began to realize if I drove, I might pass out on the way. I continued to lie in bed debating driving myself, or calling for an ambulance. Which I was leaning toward.

Eventually, in those early morning hours I finally fell asleep. Hours later, I woke feeling just a little bit better. With a new feeling. One of actually being more rested, though still quite exhausted. Possibly the effect of the low oxygen levels.

But I felt I was finally over the worst of it. As if a fever had broken. Though, I never did show a fever. In fact, my temperature was slightly lower than normal throughout the experience. As if my immune system wasn't recognizing this disease at all. Which seemed, bizarre. All I had then was a thermometer, which never showed a fever that week. This was before we knew about those finger sensors for pulse and oxygen levels.

Over the next two years, whenever I experienced COVID, I never did show a fever. I didn't have many of the usual or common symptoms we eventually heard about in the news. When people presented with COVID in the hospitals. Which was not that uncommon, I later on started to hear. This truly was a bizarre and "novel virus". A term I began to hear a lot. "Novel", as in new, unknown.

Another thing that was unusual. I never once tested positive on a COVID-19 test. At its first occurrence of course, there were none available, since no one even knew what it was, yet. I heard of people who went to the hospital only to be sent home, being told it was "just" the "flu". Nope. It was definitely not just the flu. Some then died at home. Some, in the ED waiting rooms.

By a year later I had realized two things. First, had I gone to the hospital that third night, though they may even have admitted me, as my symptoms were quite severe, they probably would have thought it was "just a flu". It was still too new. Secondly, there were people who I learned later, didn't have COVID as badly as I was presenting with, but who died waiting to see a doctor, sitting in the ED waiting room.

Even though I never tested positive, my VA doctor said that from my descriptions and events that transpired (paramedics, ED visit, etc.), he definitely believes I'd had COVID-19. To be clear about home COVID-19 tests, and again according to my doctor, if a test indicates you do have COVID-19, odds are you really do have COVID-19. But if it says you do not have it, a certain percentage of that is, or can be, incorrect.

If I remember correctly, he'd said about 20-25% can be incorrect. Even if you have it professionally done, due to timing and other issues. From the beginning, testing proved problematic. Even when performed at a hospital by a lab.

In what I know about the newer Omicron variant of COVID-19, it again all matches up to my having been infected by it. Typically, whenever I asked medical personnel for a COVID-19 test, they would simply refuse, saying it wouldn't necessarily prove anything, one way or another, and for several reasons. That was frustrating. I couldn't get a test and when I could, they saw no need for it.

Again, COVID-19 is a frustrating disease. But so is healthcare. Still, my thought at the time was that I would eventually just heal up and be done with this damn thing.

For those who berate research and medical personal over their seeming "incompetence" of COVID, it's quite obvious now that people simply did not understand either the complexity, or the variances this disease exhibits. To those angry people I'd say, "Stop being afraid, lighten up, and yes, you may needlessly die. Many have. That's life. It sucks. Moving on...it's not all the fault of our healthcare professionals. Not back then, surely."

I had all those thoughts myself over these past two years about my own situation. Yeah, it sucks! But you do what you can and if and when you can, you move on. I remember many times, thinking, "I can't go out THIS way! Not like THIS! Dying alone? In bed. At home? Not plummeting to the earth in a plane with my hair on fire...or some other magnificent death? No!"

After all the more rewarding ways I had opportunities to die from over my lifetime (car racing, sky diving, climbing, SCUBA, motorcycles, bodyguard, even just being IN the USAF, and so on). But THIS? This, just wasn't acceptable! There are so many frustrations involved with COVID.

By Thursday of my first week with COVID-19, I felt well enough to finally do some laundry and wash my bed sheets. Which meant I had to go downstairs to my basement. Ten steps. It's TEN steps on those stairs. I got my sheets, took my time walking downstairs, being careful as I felt weak. I started the wash. Then came back up those same ten steps. By now I was breathing hard. I sat back down in my living room recliner.

I have never before had a recliner in my entire life. When I moved in here, it was just here. So when the professional rug cleaner cleaned the rugs (which we ended up replacing), I had him clean the recliner, too. I'm so glad I did. For COVID alone, if for nothing else.

I sat there catching my breath for nearly fifteen minutes before breathing returned to normal. I was surprised by that. Normally it wasn't a problem. Not at all. I did not then realize, or even know about those issues with COVID and low oxygen levels.

Or that it was leading some victims to experience serious damage. Sometimes damaging organs beyond all repair. Damage that eventually killed some people in killing parts of their brain. Or heart, as I referenced earlier regarding PET scans of the inner heart muscle tissues. (see ref# 7)

As I said, my VA doctor had me take plenty of tests over the past two years. So I really can't complain. It appears however, that (somehow) I'm fine. Somehow I escaped serious COVID damage. So far anyway. However, only time will really tell us what the long term damages are. Still, as it is, things are promising.

Blood Clotting & The Venous Pulmonary System

With COVID, we have seen some issues with blood clots, the thickening of blood, and even alterations of one's veins. They have found "pillars" generating within veins and vesicles due to COVID. Which no one ever seems to mention in research I've surveyed. Yet, I did find a paper on it: "COVID-19 is a systemic

vascular hemopathy: insight for mechanistic and clinical aspects."
More about that in a moment. (see, ref# 8)

Consider this, that you may not know about our veins:

> "A human being's vessels likely undergo slight damage on a
> daily basis, she said. Sitting in one position for a long time,
> or carrying a heavy bag on your shoulders, for instance, can
> slightly squeeze or compress blood vessels. But the body
> can respond easily to these minor injuries by increasing
> levels of Atf3 and, in turn, regenerating the cells around
> injured vessels. There is a point, though, when the damage
> is too extensive or where cells are older and aren't
> responding as well," Said, Luisa Iruela-Arispe" PhD. Chair,
> Department of Cell and Developmental Biology. Stephen
> Walter Ranson Professor of Cell Biology (see, ref# 9)

After having contracted COVID and beginning to heal from it, I
started noticing what I could only believe were random and
infrequent clotting issues in my veins and blood vesicles. I
noticed discomfort in my head, forehead, scalp, and other places.
Weirdly, very specifically located "headaches". I could tell (or
believed) that it was in a single vein. It was odd.

I also noticed this over the next year and in very specific locations
in my calves and feet. I would rub my feet, especially the ball of
my foot, until I got the blood moving again. Sometimes I would
take an 81mg aspirin and it would clear up. Although I was
concerned about a clot dislodging, traveling to my brain and
giving me a stroke.

A few years previously, my doctor had suggested my considering
taking a daily 81mg aspirin as a preventative heart health measure
due to my age. It had long been pretty standard when you hit a
certain age. I agreed for a couple of years until in 2022 the
USPSTF suggested we stopped doing that as a mere precaution,

due to one's age. Unless you have an actual issue. These new findings said it wasn't worth the potential of intestinal bleeding. (see, ref# 10) So I had stopped. My still taking that daily aspirin at the time of my initial bout with COVID, may well have saved my life. The stats kind of prove it.

I wasn't sure what was going on with these blood clots, until I read about people with COVID experiencing similar blood clotting:

> "'Some people infected with SARS-CoV-2 develop abnormal blood clotting. In some with COVID-19, we're seeing a massive inflammatory response, the cytokine storm that raises clotting factors in the blood,'" says Galiatsatos, who treats patients with COVID-19." (see, ref# 11)

So? Had I experienced a cytokine storm? I noticed that first week of COVID that it was affecting my entire venous system. It felt like a weak solution of Draino being run through my system. Like acid in my veins.

I later came to realize, all along the inside of all my veins, arteries and vesicles, the interior surfaces were being irritated and inflamed. I also realized, for the first time in my life, that I could literally feel all my veins. Or it felt that way. Which was to say it was at the very least, disturbing. At the most, rather frightening.

I started finding bizarre medical papers on this. The most curious for me was on, "pillars". (see, ref# 11). As best I understand it, there are several issues and explanations. Either the virus, or our own immune system, attacks the inner surfaces of our veins, heart muscle, arteries, etc. That's one issue. Recent research, as I previously mentioned, indicates we can "see" damage to muscle cells on the inside of the heart using a PET scan. Cells that cannot be regenerated, which is ominous. (see ref# 7)

Another issue are those "pillars". Apparently when a vesicle or vein (I'll just refer to "vein" for all sizes of them) is broken, they can reattach by growing toward one another and rejoining. Good. That's normal. That is I would assume, the "pillar" growing function.

A vein is a tube after all, or a kind of pillar, if you like. So a vein's circumference grows forward to reattach to its other detached section, growing all the way around as a tubule, or pillar, and hopefully fully reattaches itself. Apparently, this is a not infrequent and natural occurrence. Our system healing/repairing itself.

However, if this function is fundamentally tampered with, as in a virus infecting cells in a vein, a pillar can grow anywhere from, in, or on a vein. Even in a cross section of the vein, from one side to the other. Or from one vein to another adjacent vein located nearby, joining the sides of two veins not previously joined. Research on this indicated they had not yet seen this being a problem.

That surprised me. As a pillar traversing a vein inside, would seem to allow for a blockage of blood cells. Which could potentially lead to problems. But they indicated that hasn't been the case in macrophages gone wild, allowing a back up/blockage of blood transported cells within veins. Well, good to know.

> "Macrophages can grab the broken ends of a ruptured blood vessel in the brain and 'stick' them back together, helping them heal faster." Also, "Microbleeding occurs very often in the human brain, particularly in elderly people," says Dr. Luo Lingfei, a developmental geneticist at Southwest University." (see, ref# 12)

Getting back to blood clotting. I had experienced this from time to time over the first year or so of COVID, in various parts of my body, as I mentioned. I have a heavy foot-massager floor device my sister gave me a while back, as she never used it. I had the idea to use that to break up the clots in my feet, typically in the ball of my foot. I have flat feet, they're sore sometimes, so it was kind of fun and pleasing to use from time to time. But mostly I found I had little use for it also.

I would with COVID at times notice that ball of my foot would become cold. I assumed, due to clotting action. Heat also helped to alleviate the issue. As would the 81mg aspirin, in my "nuclear option" if need be. I worried about sitting so much for months. Blood needs to move more than normal and regularly, we need a goodly amount of exercise on a daily basis.

The pain I felt from this clotting action was typically in my calves, or my head, just above my eyes. Which concerned me the most. A clot forming there could lead to a stroke, and I took that very seriously.

Also, sometimes my (typically right) calve would ache, always in the same specific location. I could usually hand massage it and the issue would go away. But that concerned me too as again, a broken up clot in one's blood stream could block a vein elsewhere. In the heart, or the brain. While aspirin might would affect the entire blood system related to a clot. And a massage/breaking up of a clot, wouldn't.

The 81mg of aspirin I assumed always worked the best, in thinning the blood. Luckily, this wasn't a situation I had very often. But happening at all, or ever, still felt like it was far too often.

Air Quality and Breathing

I have lived in the Pacific Northwest for most of my life. The past few years, as many states have, we've had bad climate change, forest wildfire, air quality issues. So, I thought I should mention something about, breathing and air quality. I'll skip most of what I went through and go right to last night, as I write this (Sunday, October 9, 2022).

I woke at 2AM with high blood pressure symptoms. Not bad ones, but I could feel my pulse all though my body, which was pretty uncomfortable. I checked air quality ("Alexa, what's the air quality in Bremerton"). It was "unhealthy" at 101 on the index. Not so good. So I got up, drank some water, unusually took an entire Benadryl and went back to bed.

Lying back in bed, the Benadryl worked a little, but it wasn't working well enough. I got back up and put on a COVID mask, then went back to bed. That did help and I fell back asleep. Had it not been for the pandemic, I wouldn't normally have had such a mask to put on. But then, I probably would not have had these symptoms, either.

I woke again feeling better at 4AM, better than when I woke at 2AM. Air quality was also a little better and down into the high end of moderate, around 90. I fell back asleep and woke again at 6AM. Air quality was now a bit lower at 81. I got up, took off the mask and brushed my teeth, etc. By time I got to the kitchen to make an espresso and breakfast, I started not feeling very good at all.

I was very confused as to what to do. I made some Tulsi tea (allegedly good for the vagus nerve (see, ref# 73), rather than my usual espresso, and fried two eggs with no salt, just butter. That, rather than eating a frozen, pre-made breakfast with higher than needed sodium levels. I ate, drank my herbal tea, watched some news on TV and continued to deteriorate in as much comfort as possible.

Finally, I put the mask back on. Within five to ten minutes, I felt better. As I had skipped a night on taking CBDs at bedtime, I had taken them the night before, but only a half dose (like a quarter dropper full). I was worried that I wasn't responding well to them.

But with the mask showing much improvement, it led me to the judgment that it was probably air quality affecting me so poorly. So I kept it on. If all I have to do until the air gets better around here is to wear a mask, I'm just fine with that.

I checked air quality again at 8:45AM. It was slightly higher, at 84. I kept the mask on and kept hydrating (that's also necessary). It's important to recognize what's actually affecting you and respond appropriately.

I had worried around 4AM that I might need to call paramedics again. I really didn't want to. IF they came, what could they do? Give me oxygen? I was getting air. It was just poisoned with forest fire smoke. Which can be pretty toxic. Even more so when there are structures being burned and not just trees.

This became yet another health delay in finishing this book. On Monday, air quality was moderate but still giving me issues. I figured I'll just be wearing a mask until I don't have to. Maybe Tuesday? Will I have to sleep with it again that night? It's suppose to clear up this week but return on Friday. I can't help but wonder/worry about others who are going through this. Or far worse.

> On exposure to smoke from fires: "Smoke can contain many different chemicals, including aldehydes, acid gases, sulfur dioxide, nitrogen oxides, polycyclic aromatic hydrocarbons (PAHs), benzene, toluene, styrene, metals and dioxins." - Dept of Health (see, ref# 13)

Be aware of your surroundings. It may not just be the disease, LC, or whatever you've been eating or drinking. Though LC may make you hyper sensitive to things or magnify the effects of things. For now, we have to be creative in managing the condition. What we breathe can indeed affect us when we're in a very sensitive state.

COVID-19 Symptoms

Examples of common symptoms of Long Covid include (my symptoms in bold):

- **Tiredness or fatigue (it was strange waking, after even a good night's sleep, still feeling tired, or "exhausted")**

- **Difficulty thinking or concentrating (sometimes called, "brain fog")**

- Shortness of breath or difficulty breathing (I had this once, that was really noticeable)

- Headache (not as many were experienced, until my BP problems in an unusual headache)

- **Intermittent high blood pressure**

- Dizziness on standing

- **Intermittent fast-beating or pounding heart (known as heart palpitations)**

- Chest pain

- Cough (I had that only the first week in February 2020)

- Joint or muscle pain

- Depression or anxiety (I was never depressed, sometimes anxious, but LC did get to the point of my wondering in a "is this never going to end" kind of apathy, which eventually passed)

- Fever

- Loss of taste or smell

"This list is not exhaustive. Some people also experience damage to multiple organs including the heart, lungs, kidneys, skin, and brain." - From HHS.gov

Alcohol

Regarding alcohol, one of humanity's oldest medicines. I've made use of it in that way ever since I was twelve, when my grandfather told my mother to give me an old Czechoslovakian remedy called, "Schvatsky" (or, "Schvotsky"?). My mother had also been given it as a kid.

To make it, boil whiskey with bacon bits in it, along with a fresh lemon slice, honey and cayenne. Blend to desired strength, the spicier the better. No water. Drink. You quickly sweat out some, your throat is coated a bit with the honey. Lemon has long been used itself as a natural remedy.

As for the bacon? I have no idea. My older brother once said he considered the bacon as being similar to using chicken soup. Which allegedly has some useful enzymes and anti-inflammatory properties. Or something. Which bacon doesn't have, though bacon's fat and salt and flavor may offer some comforting benefits. Though bacon contains proteins, some vitamins and minerals, it lacks the nutrients and potential immune-boosting properties chicken soup is known for.

"Modern research has actually shown that chicken soup,

more than other hot liquid, increases mucus flow and helps the body rid itself of the cold virus. Chicken is rich in an amino acid called cysteine which helps loosen secretions. This effect is increased by adding spices such as pepper and garlic." - McGill, Office for Science and Society, "Separating Sense from Nonsense" (see ref# 14)

Well, that explains some of it, and the cayenne makes sense. So, from time to time I've used alcohol for illness. As many have all through history. It can also help dry you out, kill some of the pain, help you sleep. Or just act as relief for a bit from whatever miserable disease you're experiencing. If not simply numb you out.

However, with this Long Covid, I didn't dare try alcohol. Then I read in the Long Covid social media group, someone saying, "whatever you do don't drink alcohol, as it can lead to a really miserable experience." So I avoided it. When I finally did try some, I tried half a pint of Guinness. But not until I was feeling better after months suffering through LC.

It was very enjoyable to drink with lunch that day. Though by evening, I was not enjoying it so much anymore. Remember that alcohol is metabolized in the liver, and as sugar can, affects insulin levels. I mention this because alcohol and sugar became guiding elements in monitoring my healing from LC.

Another person in the social media group said it really helped him get through LC. So, that's the thing about this disease. It can be different for everyone. Just be careful. And test a little of something before jumping all in. Otherwise, you may really regret the reaction.

CBDs were another related issue. Some in the LC Facebook group said they couldn't make it without their CBDs. For me, while the had been just fine before COVID, were a nightmare for me with it.

Chapter 2

Chapter 3

My First "Long Covid"

My initial COVID symptoms, as I've said, lasted six days. Having begun on a Sunday, by that Friday I felt I was on the mend. I had no idea how long that stage (eventually morphing into "Long Covid") would last. Or even what it was that I was going through. It long felt (I long believed) that I had never mended from initial symptoms. Until I learned of LC as a kind of part two to the disease. A kind of viral Matryoshka doll inside a doll, etc.

I spent the next two years, slowly and annoyingly so, much slower than my normal speed, researching and updating my information on newer medical research. I say very slowly because I had no energy or desire and I had to force myself to look anything up on the internet.

At times I'd look something up, find it, lay back dozing off, laptop on my lap, and (especially, in the beginning) even falling asleep. Then I'd come back to it (or, wake up) and continue. It was painful, excruciatingly slow work.

Over time I began to accrue a picture of what I was going through. And it disturbed me. As in the beginning I seemed to be one of the few, of everyone I knew, who were getting a handle on what was happening. Along with medical professionals who were on top of the situation, and/or on the front lines. I was shocked to find where some medical staff were actually denying the science. Sounding political, not medical. These have been strange times, in so very many ways. And it's not over in those many ways.

I began to understand the frustration I saw from many doctors and nurses on TV news, where no one was listening. Or at times, even believing them at all. Like we were in a dream where there were massive bubbles of ignorance out there. Or at times, mere stupidity. That is, those purposely choosing to be ignorant against all reason. Some who even (and obviously) knew better, yet still refused to admit it. Utterly bizarre.

In this research I avoided pop medical sites and always looked for information from reputable research hospitals and government medical agencies. Some of whom, indeed due to toxic political influences, were actually screwing up.

It seemed we were on our own in so many ways.

I used our government as reference, but also surveyed other government's and international research hospitals. I did my best to cross-reference/cross-check and "vet" my information. So it was months before I gained any real insight to what I had been experiencing. And just what was going on inside my body. Beyond what I was directly observing myself. Society was free floating within a glut of science, confused science, experimental science and outright political mischief and amidst general paranoia.

I listened along with the rest of America, and the world, to what had happened to us. To what was happening to us all. It was a month or two then before the world really started reporting on what was happening. That was when I came to know just what I had acquired, as people in other countries around the world were dying. And then here, nation wide.

Eventually, I came to learn of that first case discovered in Snohomish county, just across the waters of Puget Sound from me here in Bremerton. Then more "first infections" occurred, at Life Care Center of Kirkland, in neighboring King County. Near to Seattle across the water of Lake Washington which I used to commute over on the 520 floating bridge, or the newer, further south I-90 floating bridge.

It was months later before I felt my lungs healed enough to feel somewhat normal again. It took months more than that before my lungs actually felt normal again. It all lasted about eight months, along with an intermittent malaise that left me in my living room recliner, day after day. Mostly just watching TV as that's all I could concentrate on, intermittently falling asleep throughout each and every day. But in the end was it eight months, or fourteen? I'll never know for sure. Was it Long Covid, or something else? Like reinfection?

I learned to use the Fred Meyer and Safeway grocery deliveries, and came to like it. It was a little more expensive, but a luxury I'd never have otherwise used. I tried shopping once, found it exhausting and perhaps, dangerous from what I was hearing and so gave ordering in a chance.

During those months I would lose time. I'd close my eyes to "rest them", then wake up minutes. or even hours later. Still feeling too tired for it to be reasonable. Especially with as much sleep as I was getting.

It was a bizarre existence. Sleep at night would be broken, with periods of being fully awake. Then, suddenly I'd fall back asleep for minutes. or hours. My sleep cycle was utterly confused. I was lucky I'm retired. I have no idea what I would have done (as many others have suffered through), had I still been in the IT work force. Though I would have been working from home and there's something in that.

I was being hit with recurring bouts of Long Covid symptoms on a monthly basis. Bouts that would last from one to three weeks (or longer), each and every month. I would have a week or two where I felt almost normal. And to add to that, after all that time feeling sick and sedentary, I knew I was becoming ever more out of shape.

For a while I would think I was getting over it, then I'd find I'd been in my recliner again, and days had passed. It was bizarre and disparaging. I could definitely see how others could become hopeless. Depressed. But I'd had a somewhat difficult childhood requiring a lot of humor and taking life as lightly as possible, when possible.

Many of those people suffering deeper and worse emotional issues than I had, were experiencing far worse symptoms than I was dealing with. If I felt I was suffering in my situation, I couldn't imagine what others must be going through. I felt for them, deeply.

By the time I had gotten over that first Long Covid, I was in the worst shape of my entire life. It was winter by then and we were approaching 2021. Typically, I have rather difficult winters anymore, anyway. Allergy problems, mostly and not enough exercising.

With Long Covid now on top of that, it became pretty confusing. Was I just having a typical difficult winter? Or was it Long Covid? Was I being paranoid, or acting like a hypochondriac? I've always been a bit paranoid about that as my mom always seemed to be sick with one thing, or another.

I was beginning now as I got older, to understand retired "snow birds" who migrated from their northern home towns to southern warmer climes during winters. I'd never much loved the cold. I always saw myself as more of a summer person. A surfer rather than a skier, you might say.

Cold just makes me want to hibernate. I used to say I thought I was part bear. But I also know the more I get out into the cold and get some exercise, the better I feel. And the lower I can keep the temperature in my house.

Still, Long Covid is nothing if not a frustrating, confusing and miserable disease.

Long Covid and Americans with Disabilities Act

Those with LC do have some legal protections. Many who have returned to work with LC, have been helped by their company so they can work in greater comfort. Either through being allowed more breaks, with those having endurance issues, or given easier jobs for a while.

Those working at say, a factory, may be given another job to do until they can return to their normal positions. A federal law covers companies with more than fifteen employees about this. For companies with fewer employees, state laws may well apply.

> "Some individuals who had COVID-19 are experiencing ongoing effects or lingering symptoms for months afterward. The scientific name for this medical condition is Post-acute COVID-19 Syndrome, or Long COVID. If you're one of the individuals who has this condition, sometimes referred to as "long haulers," you may have difficulty working in the same way you did before you had COVID-19, and you may wonder whether to ask your employer to make changes so you can do your job. Title I of the Americans with Disabilities Act (ADA) requires covered employers to make reasonable changes (referred to as "accommodations") in the workplace for qualified applicants and employees with medical conditions that meet the definition of disability.

> "Consequently, it is important to consider the definition of disability under the ADA to determine if it applies to your specific situation. The definition of disability under the ADA is broad to help ensure that people with medical conditions can work if they choose. Even if you don't think of yourself as having a disability, you may meet the ADA definition." (See, ref# 15)

Chapter 4

Omicron Variant

Contracting COVID in February 2020, I knew I had acquired a miserable and "novel" disease. I suspect I had also acquired it again later, and more than once. Between my first infection and last one, on March 28, 2022, which landed me in the emergency department for four hours. That last version was by far the worse nightmare.

Other variants around March 2022 were prevalent like the Delta variant and sub-lineages, and the Deltacron variant, a hybrid of Delta and Omicron. Whatever I had caught the second time, it was a real monster of an infection.

I thought my first COVID infection couldn't be worse. But I was wrong. I've never had issues with my heart before, which had always been strong and healthy. I'd never had any issues with my heart rate, or blood pressure. That all changed drastically as of this last infection.

I will just say here, ahead of time, what follows was my first experience (second with LC) with how LC can compromise one's vagus nerve governing the heart, heart rate/pulse and blood pressure. (see, ref# 73) It even controls our stomach and other things. I'd never even heard of this before. Now I wish I'd never had to learn of it. It took me a while before I made the connection to the vagus nerve, as being primary in the problems I had been having. (see, ref# 16)

Once I made that connection to the vagus nerve, information started flooding in. It turned out that a close relative of mine near my age (a few months younger), knew a lot about vagus nerve issues. In part, from getting off of meds after a devastating death of someone very close to her, over much of her life. Getting off fluoxetine after using it for four years, turned out to be dangerously problematic. Trust your healthcare provider...trust, but verify. An aware, informed individual can find healthcare far more safe, and useful. And therefore, life much easier.

Finally, finding health professionals who understood the drug, they've helped her ease off that medicine, which had affected her own vagus nerve. She told me that some of what I was going through from LC, she had been going through from ending that medication.

Which her doctor had put her on, but did not fully explain, or perhaps understand the ramifications himself. A medication she did need to help her through what must have felt like half of her personality being ripped away. But, some doctors believe you can safely just stop that drug. Which apparently, at least for some, or for some in using it for long enough, can be if not dangerous, feel like it is.

As she put it:

> "I was on mine [fluoxetine] for about four years and it started making me really sick to my stomach. Took me a year and a half to figure out it was the medication. And now as I'm tapering for the first couple of weeks, my belly is not too good, and I swing from depression to flying high. That all settles down in about 3 to 4 weeks. Then I wait a week and do another drop [in medication]. My first drop was just 2.6%. From 3.75 mg to 3.65. My next job I'll do next week down to 3.5. I've learned how to crush the tablets and mix with maple syrup and water to make a liquid so I can draw it out with a syringe [for gauging amount]."

She continued:

> "I'm watching a super good video made by withdrawal
> specialists in London. All about how these antidepressants
> can cause withdrawal. Also research done on chemical
> imbalance in the brain, and research is now showing that
> that's not what causes depression. The pharmaceutical
> companies have had a lot of say in this area in order to sell
> drugs. But now enough people are stepping up to the plate
> like me, and saying it's not a relapse, These are withdrawal
> symptoms and that one can get chemically dependent on
> these drugs. It's actually, really fascinating." (see, ref# 17)

On Sunday, March 28th, 2022, I thought I just had another sinus
headache. I've had many over my life time. And a few sinus
infections. I had sinus surgery back in about 1990. Which made
my life much better.

It had taken me years, not until I was an adult, that I realized I
even had allergy/sinus issues and that most of my headaches were
allergy/sinus related. Though one migraine put me in the hospital
in 12th grade for a few days.

My doctors (for some reason, three neurosurgeons) decided, after
speaking with my mother, that it was stress related my home
environment. Mostly due to my step-father, but perhaps also to do
with school all day and work at night, along with trouble
sleeping. They said I either needed to deal with things ("Here's a
single prescription to Valium 5mg"), or that I needed to move out.
Three months later I graduated high school at seventeen and did.
And my life (and health) did get better.

As an adult I realized I just needed to take some antihistamines,
maybe some decongestants, and I could carry on. I have in recent
decades, taken my doctor's advice when I get a sinus infection,
and flush with saline and wash out my sinuses. It took a while to

get used to doing that. I didn't much like it for a while. But it works very well. So, one gets used to it. I don't use the popular (and for me useless) Netti pot, but a squeeze bottle kit I get from Costco. I use a Brita filter, a lead type to filter water, heat it for nearly two minutes in my 1200 watt microwave (don't need any organisms in my sinuses), add the included packet of sodium for the purpose and flush once or twice a day. Does wonders.

My doctor made it clear that the problem occurs when your sinuses swell, closing them off. If that lasts even a day at times, bacteria grows enough that you get an infection. Keeping them open, flushing them out, ends that issue.

Antibiotics, back in the day (mostly) uselessly given for sinus infections, are now known to be even counterproductive. They dilute the effectiveness of antibiotics in general, over the entire population. Which is a dangerous thing for us all. Luckily, advances are being made on new types of drugs to take their place. Antibiotics are only good for sinus infections in an extreme situations.

> NOTE: As I'm editing this (10 Oct. 2022), a visual migraine is coming on (second in a week, and I don't get these often), which blinds me somewhat with colors, and I have to stop editing until it clears. I get these often enough now that in my daily health log I just note "MV" (migraine visuals) and take a half or whole Chlorpheniramine Maleate (CM) pill and within twenty minutes I'm fine again. However my eye doctor/surgeon recently told me it goes away in about that time anyway and maybe I should try to see what happens without taking anything. CM isn't great for you as you get older due to it's drying out effect. I need to try that, I guess. Though it is kind of disconcerting losing vision for a bit and it being replaced with colorful swirls.

Washington state is having its worst wild fire issues and the smoke has been bad of late (summer 2022). After a over a week not exercising outdoors, due to poor air quality, yesterday I got out for my typically every other day, five mile walk on my home street. The air quality was good just long enough for my walk. Today, it's worse. It's smokey, looking outside and across part of Puget Sound. Writing and editing this book has been a journey, if not at times, a trial. This has been a trial at times in having to re-read over and over, about the most difficult health experiences I have ever had. Moving on now...

When I was a kid and got a sinus infection, I was given antibiotics. So all this was an uncomfortable change for me in flushing, instead. Though, after medical professionals began warning us that we have historically been overusing antibiotics decades ago, I did stopped using them back in the 1990s. Especially for my kids when they were young, unless they were actually required.

Having had bronchitis as a kid on an almost annual basis for some years, I received antibiotics for that along with codeine cough medicine, which tasted to me as a kid like Comet cleanser, to suppress that painful and loud cough it's known for. For infections like that antibiotics are indeed useful. So when I acquired my first COVID infection, I knew what lung pain from respiratory illness felt like. But COVID presented for me, something quite different.

Omicron variant (or whatever variant it was, because it was definitely different than the first infection) was even more different, still. Certainly compared to my first and initial 2020 COVID infection. A novel, novel-virus variant, indeed. When that hit, it hit oddly enough, again on a Sunday. Sundays and 2AM were forming a pattern, at least in my mind. Weird.

I realized later that two weeks before that first day of that new infection, I'd had issues with my pulse. That was two weeks previous. Something I'd forgotten about it. I'm unsure how to explain that timeline. So I actually caught it two weeks earlier? And only later it was presenting in a more serious way? So what, it went on vacation for a bit, then hit me full on? It was, confusing.

That two weeks earlier, I had been sitting in my living room when my pulse suddenly starting escalating. It happened just after lunch and was pretty disturbing. At first I thought it was from something I had eaten. I'd had grilled fish with tartar sauce, on bread, with a slice of tomato. A seemingly harmless meal. Which the VA nurse agreed with later on. I've never had any problems with any foods, normally.

Tomatoes are in the nightshade family, along with eggplant, potatoes, and peppers. I wondered if I'd suddenly acquired an allergy to them? I ended up outside in my front yard, walking around. Hoping somehow that it would go down if I moved about.

Maybe giving my body an actual reason for a higher pulse rate. Maybe helping somehow to reset it? I didn't know, it was that or call paramedics or go to the doctor, hoping I wouldn't die on the way or something. I really didn't know.

This is something I would notice as this condition worsened over time. An almost magical belief in what was causing the symptoms, in some attempt to offer myself at least some kind of rational causation. Anything. Something, that I could latch onto as a cause and effect reason. Otherwise this disease was inexplicable and could lead to literally any condition. Like death?

I had recently bought a fingertip pulse oximeter. A devise to monitor your blood oxygen saturation (SpO2) as well as your pulse rate. I picked a few up for under twenty dollars each, when I first heard they were suggested to have around due to COVID.

So you could check/monitor your oxygen levels. I sent one each to my two adult kids. I had never used it after purchasing it, until my pulse went wild that day. I then found it extremely useful.

The previous year, my VA doctor had sent me a blood pressure monitor for our teleMed appointments. Then, if needed to I could take my own BP if not in his office when we met. Both devices became very important to me over this period of Long Covid. The finger monitor was how I knew on that day, two weeks prior, that my pulse had gone up over 140BPM.

I walked around outside that day with the O2/pulse monitor on the end of my finger, watching the pulse go up and down as I walked, or sat on the front porch stairs. Trying to divine what was going on helped. It all seemed so random, though. After about forty minutes, it finally got back down to normal.

What the hell was that, I had to wonder? By a few days later I had forgotten all about it as just some weird abnormality. I know that throughout life we can acquire allergies or lose them. I racked it up to something like that. Or maybe I had eaten something bad? It happens. Odd, but hopefully unimportant.

Until two weeks later. When it shot back up again and I ended up calling paramedics at 2AM in the middle of the night, as my pulse shot up over 160BPM. I had only ever called paramedics once before in my life, decades ago when my mother had an allergic reaction to some codeine cough medicine her doctor had incorrectly prescribed for her.

So it was hard for me to make the decision to call paramedics, just for myself. I kept hesitating, trying to not call. But finally I caved in and made that call. By time they got there, my pulse had gone back down to the normal range. Great, I just knew that would happen. It's like going to the doctor, or taking your car to a mechanic. Once you get there, everything's just fine!

Paramedics checked me out and decided I was fine. Though they did say I should probably go to the Emergency Department, and offered me a ride in the ambulance. They had my front door open as they were hesitating to leave. I could see past them to the nighttime street where the fire truck was with the ambulance behind it, in front of my house. I hoped my neighbors didn't notice. But it was 2:30AM and they had been quiet driving up.

I didn't want to deal with any charges from taking an ambulance. Even though between Medicare and VA, it might not have cost me financially, out of pocket. As it turned out, I never heard about a bill for the paramedics. So that was good to know. Still, I didn't know for sure for weeks or months if a bill would eventually arrive. But one never did. So I figured, paramedics aren't out of pocket, but perhaps an ambulance would be. I hoped never to find out.

I thought, if I could drive, I'd just drive. No ambulance. Besides, it was only two miles to the hospital. Right? So I asked if they thought I could drive myself. They said they saw no reason I couldn't, if I thought I could. So, they left, closing the door. I didn't call the VA triage nurse to see what she thought. To get her permission. Something that came back to bite me a week later.

I got in my car in the downstairs garage. I had to wait a few minutes for them to all to drive off, so I could get out of my driveway, then drove to the hospital. The one I had known for over two decades. Where I had from time to time taken my kids. It was still dark out, around 3AM. I drove over the Warren Avenue bridge, crossing the Port Washington Narrows, to East Bremerton. I turned off the road to the right where I knew the hospital was. Where was the sign indicating "H", hospital?

And...I could not find it! It's a huge hospital and yet, it had vanished? I wasn't feeling that great, or thinking that clearly, and started feeling a little faint (I never feel "faint"). I was also getting a bit anxious (I almost never get anxious). But there were also as I said, NO street signs saying, "H" or "Hospital", anywhere, as there always had been. Again, I wasn't thinking clearly, and that was becoming more obvious.

So I tried using "Siri" on my iPhone 11 (I've had that phone now for years after I left from many years with Verizon for Xfinity/Comcast, and it still seems brand new). That was the first time I tried to locate the hospital with my phone. I'd had the cell phone for a few years, but had never used that function. Frustratingly, it just kept telling me to, "Go to Silverdale". Which is the next town over, eleven miles away. What was going on?

No! I wanted THIS hospital, here! The one I've long known. I knew they had been building two new hospitals, side by side in Silverdale. But there I was, blocks (maybe a block?) from a major hospital, and it had vanished.

Finally, I pulled over to the side of the road. I tried the phone, again. Silverdale? Again? I actually screamed an obscenity in my frustration. I tried to calm down. Looked at the houses around me in that neighborhood in the dark. Finally, I decided I should just go home and see then how I felt. Maybe use my laptop to find what the hell was up. Where the damn hospital went.

But, I gave it one more valiant try. I drove down past where I had been already a couple of times. Down along the waterfront. I turned and headed back. This now seemed familiar. Until finally, I turned onto one street and... there it was! The hospital! Completely...dark. Well, that made sense. Now I know why I couldn't see it all lit up in the distance.

I drove all the way around it and even through the parking lot, looking in the ED windows. It was completely locked up, dead. I was stunned. How did a huge hospital just... stop... being? Remember, I said I wasn't thinking clearly. Which reinforced my desire now to just go home. I really had no choice. Or, I could drive to Silverdale?

By the time I got home, maybe ten minutes later, I was feeling exhausted. I did feel a bit better though. So I decided I would just go back to bed. I fell asleep within a few minutes and woke a few hours later. With, my pulse acting up again. Which was still not making sense to me.

I decided to look up the closest ED up on the computer. You know, I kind of liked when they used to more inaccurately call them an "ER", as "ED" for me anymore evokes erectile dysfunction TV adverts. Even though I suppose emergency department does make more sense than emergency room.

Anyway, I kept getting, "Silverdale", as the nearest one. So, what the hell. I got dressed and drove there. Although my heart/pulse was uncomfortable and my head didn't feel very clear. I just wasn't feeling 100% at all. I then realized some of that was just from a poor night's sleep, too much adrenaline flowing, in looking for and failing to find an ED. Or an entire hospital.

Finally, I got to St. Michael's ED. In Silverdale. I checked in, telling them what happened. They explained why I couldn't find the east Bremerton hospital. Six months previous, St. Michael's had shut down for this newly built version. I hadn't realized until they said that, that they were in any way connected.

Something I've heard recently is that they're having some regrets about shutting down the Bremerton hospital. Anyway, that explained it. Of course, all the street signs had been taken down. Instead of realizing that as I drove around in my confused state looking for the hospital, I had felt more like I was going crazy than what the more reasonable excuse was. Part of LC I've noticed is that when you're having a flare up, or an event, you aren't always thinking clearly. So proactively be prepared ahead of time. As much as you can.

That old Bremerton hospital had all its lights turned off when I found it. When normally it would have been all lit up at night and visible from just about anywhere nearby. But that was seven months ago when it was still open, when I'd last had lunch at their cafeteria with a friend.

I sat in that ED waiting area for about forty minutes. I was then ushered into a room and hooked up to monitors. They took blood and sent it off to run tests. A doctor came in and asked some questions. After that I just lied there for a while. At one point, I asked the nurse for a COVID test. But I got the same response I'd been getting from healthcare professionals for a while. It wouldn't be useful because of this or that reason. I wondered, why then do they keep mentioning everywhere to get a test done? If no one would give me one?

Occasionally, a nurse would check in on me, assuring me of the situation. Finally, the doctor came back and reviewed my blood tests. They showed nothing wrong with me. Oh, really? This was also something I would hear time and again. And had been, since my first COVID infection. The ED doctor had them put a two week, ZIO Patch heart monitor on me, and then they just sent me home. I felt...underwhelmed. Tired. Confused.

That two weeks...was a trial. Wearing that patch. You couldn't get it wet. You had to try not to sweat too much. You didn't want to corrode the electrodes, pressing against your skin. I was afraid to even take a shower for that first week. I didn't want to compromise the recordings. I badly wanted to know those results. Finally after a few days, honestly nearly a week, and being very careful (even a bit paranoid), I got my shower. And boy if that didn't feel incredible!

When I got home that first day with the patch I started researching in earnest. Why was this happening? I assumed it had to be COVID. Though I had seemed to be affected by whatever it was that I was eating that day. Had I suddenly become hyper sensitive to some food? All food? Was it too much salt/sodium? Or what?

Research over those next weeks and months proved interesting. As some of those concerns were indeed what seemed to be going on. Or, were they? That first day, a Monday, I had very little to eat. Fearing anything I ate would trigger another tachycardia event. Which as I discovered, exhibited in very uncomfortable ways. So I had a only couple of hard boiled eggs that first day.

That entire week I ate very little. As far as it being the "COVID diet", in the end I got down from about 225lbs to 213lbs. Felt great as far as that. So some benefits. I started off with very plain foods, adding a bit at a time as I became more comfortable with what I ate, which appeared safe.

Oddly enough, a week after that first "attack", and for the third time in two years (with first infection hitting on a Sunday, in February 2020), this time it happened on Sunday, March 28th, 2022. That next Sunday, a week later my Blood Pressure issues began and the pulse issues seemed to fade.

I got out my BP monitor and started checking my Blood Pressure. I went to bed that night and woke about 1:30AM with a headache. From high BP I learned, a new and bizarrely unpleasant feeling.

I got up, tired, frustrated and took my blood pressure. It was high at 168/88. I looked it up on the internet, on WebMD, or some other mostly reliable site. It indicated if it got up to over 160, call 911. I monitored for about twenty minutes but it had gone lower. Not to normal though. Until it finally. It hit 161 and I could feel how uncomfortable that was again, making me even more nervous.

So regretfully (while thinking, "Not again!"), I finally called 911. After the 911 operator notified paramedics, the operator stayed on the line with me until I felt more secure. I continued monitoring my BP and sharing it with her. I was feeling pretty emotionally raw by this point. Embarrassingly so, but I put that to the side for now.

After two years of this stupid COVID nonsense, after a week of seriously concerning issues in an area (my BP) that I was thoroughly unfamiliar having, I was feeling pretty vulnerable. I wanted to hang up. But to be honest, I felt better with her on the phone. She repeatedly said that was, "OK". That's how disturbing this can be when you're tired, in the middle of the night, in an unusual situation that shakes your nerves to the core and, especially when you live alone. It was all very strange.

It wasn't long before the paramedics arrived. Maybe ten minutes? Maybe, eight? Same guys, too. I mentioned they'd been there a week ago and they remembered it. I apologized, saying this was the second time in my life I called paramedics, and both within the same week.

They brushed off my concerns (and embarrassment) and checked me out. By then, I was looking pretty good, again. So why did I have to call them? Because? Better safe than sorry. Right? Better "red" (embarrassed), then dead. Maybe?

The paramedics assured me I had done the right thing. Again, they suggested I go to the ED and again, offered my the ambulance. Again, I declined. I said I would call the VA nurse and see what she thought. They said that was a good idea (she had my history available), so they packed up and headed out.

I sat there in stunned disbelief. I gathered myself and called the VA nurse. She reviewed my record and call from the previous week. Then she talked to me for an entire hour. In the end, she decided I was probably good for the night and didn't need the ED this time.

One thing I learned about all this reminded me of my first time as a parent. When I had my first, a young child who needed a hospital and I was fighting panic and anger against anyone in my way to get my kid to a doctor in the middle of the night. Humans are tougher than we think. But especially apparently, kids.

Parents with a second child don't panic quite so easily. My first emergency, middle of the night visit to the ED for my first child, had me in a state of mind of finding help my kid, or else! My young son had a high fever with extenuating circumstances. The health insurance nurse on the phone said take him the the ED.

Which was a long way away. Twenty miles. Driving in the dark, alone with my kid, while my wife and other child we're back at home. I got him in the car and drove him to Seattle from our home in Auburn, to the hospital where he'd been born. Where our insurance had long been when I worked running the mainframe from and for radiology and pathology at UWMC and, also for our regional HMC trauma center.

I carried him unconscious into the ED. A doctor met me as I entered the department and we talked. He said, "I'm sorry, but you'll have to take him to Group Health Cooperative/ Central Hospital. I was stunned. I was here now at an ED, so...HELP HIM! I was angry.

The doctor was taken aback for a moment. Then he did something disconcerting. He smiled. Then he asked, "Is this your first child?" Realizing something was up, maybe I was even over-reacting (but HOW?), I said, "Yes. Why?" He continued smiling his thankfully kind, understanding smile.

"He'll be fine, you have plenty of time. Just drive over there because that's where your health insurance is now. Right?" I thought about it. I guessed he was right. But if my son died, I'd be back.

I had indeed changed my health insurance after I left working for the University of Washington recently, where I'd worked for over seven years. Suddenly, I felt stupid. He assured me again, very kindly, just to relax. I left and got him to the other hospital, really only a few minutes away. In the end he was fine. In fact, once I got him into an exam room, the doctor found nothing wrong with him. Not even a fever. Which apparently, had broken. Of course. Remember? When you go to the doctor or take your car to a mechanic, everything is just fine. Heavy sigh...

For myself since childhood, I've had stitches multiple times. As an adult, I'd even driven myself to the hospital to get patched up. But never anything like what I was experiencing with COVID. And certainly not at this age. Which is why I liked to say that old age really isn't for the young. At times, not even for the old, if you ask me.

I had ended the call with the VA nurse about my blood pressure issues, and since I wouldn't be going to the hospital, I went back to bed. Then over the next few weeks and months, was when things got interesting...

Chapter 5

OMICRON Long Covid

It's pleasant now to note that my LC activated virus, from a COVID infection, has as of this writing, dissipated quite a bit from those first weeks. It's been gone (or very low) for weeks now and seems to be decreasing over time. Which I believe is thanks to many of the things I'm detailing here in this book. Regular exercise, diet changes, vitamin C, and proper meds, as needed.

[Note: I'm revising this book at the end of December 2023. I still have Long Covid, but it is very light now, nearly gone in its "half-life" type of ever decreasing into non-existence.]

The LC activated virus felt like a "humming", or "buzzing" all throughout my nervous system, and veins. Now, there is an overall dull "fuzzy", or "cotton-like" feeling. But not all the time. Which is nonetheless annoying and indicative of Long Covid still being there. But that's far more acceptable than that electric buzz feeling. Which had an electrochemical feel to it, and was usually too intense to want to put up with. Though, it's not like one had a choice.

I would note however, that some antihistamines (specifically for me, Benadryl) seemed to alleviate my discomfort along with antivirals (again, this worked for...me), like Valacyclovir. After a time on it, it did seem to make it feel as if LC had gone away. So for me Valacyclovir was a miracle drug. Though it may not have been he LC but this underlying, triggered virus.

Apparently this was true for others also. As that's how I came to realize it was useful. My own experiences with it before reading about it, were haphazard. As LC is so intermittent and confusing. Like it's purposefully messing around with you.

Regarding meds like Valacyclovir, COVID vaccines and boosters:

> "Since aciclovir and the later drugs Valacyclovir (Valtrex) and famciclovir (Famvir) only target these herpes viruses, it is OK to have the herpes medication and COVID vaccines at the same time. You don't need to tell the people at the vaccine centre that you are taking antivirals." From, Herpes Viruses Association's, Marian Nicholson, HVA Director (see, ref# 3)

Valacyclovir doesn't care about underlying Long Covid issues. It doesn't deactivate whatever virus that had been activated. Assuming here a probable activation of a dormant herpes virus, which most of us have. It is estimated 87.4% of 14 to 49 year olds are infected with HSV-2 but have never received a clinical diagnosis. (see, ref# 67)

Still, it does seem to relieve symptoms. Which made life livable to the point that after a week or two on the drug, it really didn't feel anymore like I had anything at all. Though some of that might be the pleasure of a decrease in discomfort, somewhat masking what was still there. But I didn't care. I mean, so what?

To me, when that first happened, it was life-changing. But it didn't fool me. I knew it was still there, hiding, or masked in some way. I knew Valacyclovir wasn't killing LC, just an activated virus sitting on top of the condition. Which was an initial bone of contention and confusion between my primary care VA doctor and myself.

Until I made it clear that I did not think Valacyclovir was ending LC. Merely decreasing the virus it had activated. For a while I just kept hearing how the literature does not indicate Valacyclovir does anything toward ending LC. Hey? Look, who cares? I just wanted to be able to get through the day. And it helped!

The only problem was my VA doctor, who understandably wasn't up-to-date on all this, lacked the information I was coming across in my pointed, motivated and time unrestricted research. Just as most physicians had not been up to date during COVID-19 and in LC's initial year or two.

After all, I was retired. My time was my own (luckily). And I was highly motivated. That is, whenever I had the energy or wasn't feeling too ill. I had all the time I needed to read all the cutting edge info I could get my eyes upon in not being a busy, overworked doctor.

My doctor eventually relented saying he's not a research doctor. They weren't a research hospital. So while we as victims may even actually know exactly what may be best for us, our doctors frequently nowadays, will remain for a while longer, unaware of that information.

Probably, for quite some time. Unless you're lucky enough to have a Long Covid research study or response team available to help you. I still do not know why there was (is?) not a VA/LC team nationally available to all those of us who were in their care.

Rules of COVID-19 and/or Long Covid

These are just from my own experiences:

1. COVID-19 has a variety of presentation formats.

    1. While a lab test is best, and home tests are useful, you or even better your doctor, can diagnose its existence from symptoms. A "clinical diagnosis" without labs, as opposed to a "differential diagnosis" with them. I say this because I've never gotten a positive home test and doctors/hospitals have refused me testing for a variety of reasons. And so my VA doctor assures me it's obvious I've had COVID-19 (and Long Covid, and most likely both) at least twice.

2. Just when you think you have it figured out, LC skews inconsistently and makes things more confusing.

3. Just when you think you're over LC, or it seems to be decreasing, it comes back and plays intermittent/ inconsistent, adding to the confusion.

4. Long Covid doesn't usually end one day, as COVID primary does. It seems to fade over time. Slowly. Very (too) slowly. Then one day you'll notice, it has just gone away. I've had it at least twice. First time having begun in February 2020. That being said, my first LC experience lasted just over a year. I hear some doctors saying it tends to last a couple of years. We're still learning, it's still too new. But having had it go away for me once already, does offer me hope for this second time.

5. Long Covid can appear to give one spontaneous, disturbing (scary), temporary food allergies that may actually be due to eating foods with sugar, and/or high histamine levels, which may evoke an intense histamine response. While this could just be coincidental, it may appear to be a food allergy.

6. Know when to back off. But try to do what you can, a bit more each day.

   1. Follow your "gut". Yes, you'll make mistakes. But in making those mistakes you are learning things. You will progress to getting better. Both in the attempts you are making, and in those attempts making you healthier. But be smart about it.

7. Be Positive! Attitude, accounts for a lot. Never let hopelessness take over or it will take you down. This disease does not deserve to live. YOU do!

Chapter 6

Remedies?

Regarding medicine, vitamins supplements and remedies. COVID-19 and LC are both only a few years old. Remember, it was only widely discovered in 2020. We're learning more about them on a daily basis. Research is ongoing and world wide.

I had quickly discovered I would have to do my own research. There's so much conflicting information, especially in its beginning, you just had to take your best "educated" guess. And if you didn't have one, you needed to set yourself up to have one. For many (including myself too often), it was a frustrating and fruitless experience. Until I acquired enough knowledge that it could build on itself. Just beware popular beliefs without evidence. Personal anecdotes are useful, but can be dangerous.

A social media group for LC sufferers was helpful on a few levels. Though not so much for remedies and medicines. Which were actually what I was there looking for. But great for emotional support in finding just how many others were ever so much worse off than I.

I found I really didn't have that much to complain about. Which put me somewhat in my place, but also left me at odds in my own misery. What I had wasn't that bad compared to others. But I was still entirely miserable.

For the past two years, I researched until I exhausted finding anything new or useful. Much of which was useless that first year or two. Findings continued to change in orientation and information. So I stopped for a while. Many were complaining about how badly this research was going on. Some even pathetically politicized and weaponized all of that. Not useful.

But that's science and medicine. We learn as we go. As new

information is made available, we update it as often as we can. Which is vastly better than wide speculation and snake oil fixes.

When LC seemed to have ended for me the first time, I stopped researching. It was a relief. But then it would come back as it hadn't ended. The worry was if I had caught it again, or not. I would return to searching for the newest information, often coming again across old information, slowing the process, in an inevitable part of research that one does their best to diminish.

After a few times of that LC cycling, I just kept researching as I could, as I had the energy and motivation. Whenever I heard of something new in the news or my news feeds, I'd dig into it again. Medical sciences finally are making some progress as we've had a couple of years of this under our medical "belts".

In just the past week or so, I heard of extremely new research (see, ref# 20) which turned up findings regarding cortisol, related to LC. Whenever I find things like that, I look it up. Along with any surrounding issues I stumble upon, or that appear relevant to me, floating around in my mind, and I digest the new info. I take notes on what to research later in that case it turns out valuable. Or disregard it when it turns out not to be.

Like, what produces cortisol? Why do people with low levels seem to be the ones catching LC? Do I have or did I have a low level of cortisol when I caught it? Was it transitory? Do I have a cortisol issue? My blood tests didn't reflect that. So was it just for that, what...week? Day. Hours in that day when it was low? Was it a cortisol issue in my contracting it at all? And so on.

White Willow Bark

I really did not want to address various counters to COVID-19 or Long Covid that are popularly believed effective, as there are too many and new ones always popping up. Better we have a mindset that protects us against what is useless and unfounded other than though anecdote or hearsay.

I'd prefer to address what is proven to work, things that we know could help, though not cure, as that is in our future. Such is the case with a new popular view about white willow bark. While it does have hope as a future replacement for antibiotics, we're no where near that now. (see, ref# 83)

To be clear, there is no scientific evidence to support the claim that white willow bark can neutralize COVID-19.

As we all well know and in fact, the World Health Organization (WHO) has warned against using unproven herbal remedies for COVID-19, as they may have harmful side effects and may interfere with other medications (always check with your health official/ medical doctor, or whoever administers your medications.

I t is reasonably advisable to cautious about this article (again, see ref# 83), as it is based on a single study that has not been peer-reviewed or published in a scientific journal yet. The study only tested willow bark extract on cell samples, not on humans or animals, and did not test specifically against COVID-19.

The authors of the study also stated that their findings do not imply willow bark extract can be used as a treatment or prevention for COVID-19, and that more research is needed to confirm the safety and efficacy of the extract.

"Extract". Note that it is not advisable this is something we should create or dose ourselves, without having appropriate expert knowledge and skills. If someone claims to have those things, or says they got something from someone who claims to (or they claim that someone claims it), do be sure to verify such contentions.

Therefore, this article does not provide conclusive evidence that willow bark can neutralize COVID-19, and it should not be taken as medical advice. Please do not rely on unproven herbal remedies for COVID as they may have harmful side effects or interfere with other medications. I hope this clarifies things.

The only study that showed some antiviral effect of willow bark extract was done in "in vitro" (not in a person's body like, "in vivo"), that is in laboratory cell samples, not in humans our "out in the world", and did not test specifically against COVID-19. The authors of the study stated that their findings do not imply that willow bark extract can be used as a treatment or prevention for COVID-19, and that more research is needed to confirm the safety and efficacy of the extract. (see, ref# 84)

Therefore again, it's inadvisable to use white willow bark for COVID-19. It's better to follow official guidelines from such authoritative organizations like the WHO or your local health authorities on how to protect yourself and others from the virus. These include the obvious: getting vaccinated, wearing a mask when reasonable (or necessary), practicing physical distancing in viral environments, washing your hands more frequently during normal times and more so during outbreak periods, and avoiding crowded or poorly ventilated spaces during viral seasons.

It's best now a days with all we now know, that simple procedures like avoiding touching your face with your hands when out in public, washing your hands upon returning home, coughing or sneezing into a restrictive buffer (such as the crook of your arm when wearing an absorbent coat for instance, not a bare arm), and so on. These are easy aides to help decrease the numbers of times we acquire viruses, or share them with others, strangers, or even loved ones. Often infection is easily avoided if we simply take the time and effort.

We have to know when to trust something and when to question appropriately questions things, and how much to. Avoid the "rabbit holes" of nonsense or conspiracy. There are just too many anymore making wild speculations without enough information or actual real evidence. Who then spread that to others as founded data and peer reviewed fact when it's simply not. And that has indeed, killed people.

Look. It's not that confusing or difficult. We really just do the best we can, and then move on...

A(nother) Word of Warning:

"Self research", is what people do themselves, obviously. It's good people do that more now than ever, and have the internet for ease of access to so much information. However, for the untrained person this can get you into a lot of trouble. Many people are not actually doing, "self research". They're merely stumbling around the internet thinking they're doing research.

Finding information is not research. Just because you find seemingly relevant info, doesn't mean it's useful to you. Or even true. Just because it seems relevant, doesn't make it so. Even professional researchers can have trouble with that. People have died over this kind if ignorance in self-study/self-research. And bizarrely, some of that info is purely, purposefully misinformation. Why that is, is another course of study entirely.

I happen to have a background in research, and I'm university trained in it. I have separate from that researched medical and medicinal research throughout parts of my lifetime. So, I can reasonably say I'm not an ordinary "layman" or "self-researcher".

Which doesn't mean I'm 100% to be trusted either. No single individual is. Which is what "peer reviewing" is all about. I am neither a doctor or a professional "medical" researcher. That being said, my studies over my lifetime have been repeatedly proven to be pretty accurate, and I've worked hard to be careful about it.

Why that is, is a long story. In part in my having been a senior technical writer, and in having achieved the high levels at which I had worked, whenever I had to research something and turn it into my managers, if I were proven wrong I wouldn't long have worked in that career, or industry.

If nothing else, using the tried and true journalistic method of "triangulation" is very useful. (see ref# 19) Something so often today with our 24 hour news cycles and instant news media environments has gone by the wayside, and far too often. Even by professionals. So "vet" your sources using other sources.

> "'Vetting', is the process of thoroughly investigating an individual, company, or other entity before making a decision to go forward with a joint project." (from, Investopedia)

Whenever you find something new and interesting (and not just seemingly relevant), check it with at least three DISPARATE sources. Trusted, reliable sources who are unrelated, even holding opposing views, which can be the strongest. Finding some small unknown blogger who agrees with you, isn't reliable just because you found an agreeing view. That's in general caused us all immense issues now a days.

When enemies or opposing ideologies agree, you may be onto something. But also use verifiable, proven sources, widely known and accepted to be reliable (don't just listen to those who may be their political enemies). Remember that whenever some information fits your beliefs a little too well, don't necessarily trust it. Trust, but verify it, and even more so. Other related background research can also help to solidify the suitability and viability of your info.

All that being said, as with anything I come up with here, one should go through their doctor about it first before trying it. We're all different and your doctor knows best how you are. They should, anyway. We should trust our educated and trained, medical professional. Especially if we know them well and have received good practices from, them over time.

Even they will tell you they "practice" medicine through their entire lives. However sometimes a person knows themselves and their body better than anyone else. I know I've run into that with previous doctors over my own lifetime.

Don't be too afraid to speak up if you think a doctor has either misdiagnosed you or misprescribes for you. Talk to them, and if need be get a second opinion. That's where peer reviews come in as that is a kind of peer review. When you find at least one other professional who agrees with a prognosis, if nothing else it can lend you assurance and that's important when going into any course of treatment for a malady.

It's a tenuous relationship and one we have to be aware of. To allow our medical professionals to help us and to help educate us. While we should not obfuscate or obstruct our medical care, any good medical professional should appreciate an informed client. Or "patient", if you prefer. Though for some that implies a "victim" mentality which can hamper growing healthy again.

Just be aware, no medical professional wants a "know-it-all" for a client. Especially, if they're closed minded. Or often wrong, or misinformed.

Regarding Cortisol

Be aware there are supplements proven to reduce cortisol, a stress hormone. In excess it can often cause physical and mental health problems. People taking vitamins/supplements, can at times cause more harm than the good they are hoping to generate. Again, it's always good to talk to your doctor(s) who know what your medical & medicinal situation is, when considering taking a new supplement, herb or drug of any kind. (see also, ref# 20)

Eliminating Potential Irritants

When I got hit with my last bout of COVID and then contracted Long Covid (again), I immediately eliminated all food for a day or so, trying to get a handle on why my body seemed to be rejecting food and reacting so poorly to what I was eating.

I immediately eliminated all sugar. Though I normally don't add sugar to food anyway. For many years I have seldom kept sugared foods and sweets around. I also eliminated all caffeinated drinks, or foods. Except coffee and tea and limited my intake to one a day.

I eliminated all vitamin supplements for a few days. Especially, if I found contraindications regarding heart issues. That included my B12, D3 (both indicted by my doctor, due to low levels on my blood tests), and glucosamine/chondroitin (for my knees, suggested by an Orthopedic joint specialist).

Glucosamine/chondroitin caused me other issues near the end of this bout of LC, taking a few weeks to negatively affect me after starting it again. So I stopped it when I realized it was my only recent change. Perhaps because of not getting enough exercise. But it was causing pain in my finger tips and down my arm, both of which stopped almost immediately when I stopped taking it. This after years of using it normally with no issues.

I rather quickly went back to my one-a-day vitamin and the B12, as I felt I needed them for overall health. And I needed the energy. There seemed to be no issues with them after starting them again, so I kept it up.

I even stopped my prescribed nightly Atorvastatin (for high

cholesterol). When my doctor said I could (should actually) go back on it, I did. That was after blood and medical tests were performed and evaluated. Also, be very careful about stopping any prescribed medicine, even a statin. I immediately told the nurse I was stopping my statin, who told me it should have no imminent danger in stopping it. But should mention it to my doctor next time we spoke or I communicated with him.

What's important here is not necessarily what I was taking. But how I handled the situation when I contracted COVID-19/LC. I spoke with a medical professional first, and researched to find any potential issues in between my heart and these supplements.

 Stopping them, even the ones my doctor had suggested (not ordered), I then told my doctor, and tested out starting to take them again. If there were issues (there weren't for me), I'd then stop and contact someone.

Vitamin Supplements

As with any of this kind of thing, it never hurts to run things by your doctor (have I said this enough yet?). They really are there for us. Though sometimes it may just not feel like it. Push through that. As sometimes it can merely be a misperception. Or their attention needs to be better acquired properly.

MELATONIN (temporary supplement): Proven for me for years for sleep when needed. But I only use 5mg (I understand you only need 3mg), only on nights when it's very necessary and I tend to break a tablet in half. So I use it as little as possible, trying instead to get enough sunlight for at least fifteen minutes a day (when it exists here in the PNW)

Better to avoid needing melatonin supplements. Consider, the more one takes melatonin, the less the body thinks it needs to produce it. So it can, as so many drugs/supplements can do, cause a self-perpetuating loop.

GABA (temporary supplement): I wanted to look into this for sleep issues. I'd tried various supplements that help with enhancing mental processes, but they all make it hard for me to sleep at night, even if they did aid thinking. Melatonin had often been the answer before when it was hard to sleep. But again, I try not to use it for long term. GABA was suggested by my brother who is a very smart guy. So if it works, I'll research it's long or short term use, even more.

However, I found as I became more normal, getting over LC I could sleep better on a regular basis. It may even have been the triggered dormant virus. Inability to sleep, helped point out to me that I was having some kind of issue or another that I needed to address (i.e., LC returning, getting stronger, more energy, a lack of enough sunlight, etc.).

Valacyclovir, 500mg (typically a temporary medicine): Through LC, this was a life saver for me. Though generally a temporary medicine, usually for three, or five days (though for some extreme cases doctors have prescribed long term daily use). It is indicated in some medical literature as being used at times for Long Covid viral activation of a dormant virus.

Remember that there are other forms of the virus aside from the more well known oral, or genitals herpes as with chickenpox or shingles. Long Covid apparently makes use of that by activating a dormant virus, which is in part why there are so many potential symptoms. (see ref# 20)

From, Very Well Health:

> "The viruses at play here mainly fall under the Herpes viridae family. Most Americans carry a dormant version of herpes viruses. An estimated 87.4% of U.S. adults aged 14 to 49 years infected with HSV-2 remain asymptomatic with no clinical diagnosis. Likely over 95% of adults carry

Epstein-Barr virus (EBV). After our immune system defeats any virus in the herpes virus family, that virus will burrow into our nerves and go into a dormant (latent) state." (see, ref# 21)

VITIMAN C schedule of use (temporary supplement, normal inclusion within diet): I found a reference in a standard doctor's prescription being used (see, ref# 22) that uses 1,000mg, 5 times a day for a week for an LC herpes virus activation. Then 1,000mg with each meal (I added one at bed time) for three days. I then went with just 1,000mg with each meal until no longer needed.

This comes from medical research where they found the Herpes virus does not seem to like Vitamin C very much. My thought was that if this helped with outbreaks, it might help with a Long Covid reactivation. And it did seem to help. A lot. (see, refs# 11 & 12) Vitamin C use for alleviation of some diseases does warrant some care, as too much can give you some side effects.

One doctor warned me that taking Vitamin C for all disease issues could potentially even help not just your immune system, but also the actual disease. However, I've not been able to find any documentation or examples of that today. His contention was, we may not yet know if that can be the case, so don't overuse it. (see ref# 23) There has been a decades long health supplement culture belief in mega-dosing Vitamin C. I have not myself recently researched where that debate is at today.

PANTOTHENIC ACID (temporary supplement) as related to cortisol production: I acquired some, but haven't really tried it yet. The trouble is, some of these things can react on me rather (very) poorly. So trying new things now (something I've never shied from all my life), feels very tenuous. And frankly, nothing says it would work. It was just of potential use and a presupposition from some research on those who caught LC, in having had low cortisol levels. Some information even indicates cortisol issues may be questionable. (see, ref# 20)

ZINC, Zn (temporary supplement) as related to cortisol production: Also as useful in fighting colds/flu. Zink is an inhibitor of HSV replication in vitro; its effect in vivo is to enhance cell-mediated immunity. (see, ref# 22) My experience at the writing of this book is that it was making me very uncomfortable for some reason. Some information even indicates too high of a dose can be bad for you. (see, ref# 20)

HERBAL TEAS (diet): Reasonable herbal teas, can't hurt. Some unreasonable ones can. I've been using TULSI TEA (Organic India brand). Recommended by some for vagus nerve issues. My doctor said he had never heard of that, but then there was much other he hadn't heard of, yet. TUMERIC TEA (Organic India brand): The two I've been using daily are, Tulsi Tumeric Ginger tea and Bigelow Ginger Peach Tumeric. I've been using these because they are available to me in my local stores, are reported to have a calming effect, and aid the health of the vagus nerve. And I like their taste best. I first tried a rose hips Tulsi tea which I found personally having far too much of a cloying taste.

ANCIENT CHINESE HERBAL MEDICINES: I've used these in the past under the care of a practitioner with years of experience and was amazed at their benefit. I did not use this during my COVID-19/LC experience though I have used them for allergies and other things in the past. I do prefer herbs over western medicine where possible, as they tend to be less harsh and gentler on your system. If not at times more effective. Western meds are amazing when needed and used correctly. But can also frequently be overkill. I found years ago that I do better with half doses of prescriptions. That's mostly, with pain meds, but with many meds the smallest functional dose that works is better than too big of a dose in what is being recommended. I also stop using them as quickly as possible. This is a problematic contention. While some drugs need a certain dose to be most effective, there are indeed times where it's western medicine overkill. Trust, but verify. Ask your doctor. They are usually reasonable and if you want to use less, they'll tell you when that's reasonable or why it's not.

UNLESS however, it is something like antibiotics in which case, it's always best to follow doctor's orders, always. And always finish the prescription as prescribed. To do otherwise can lead to antibiotics becoming less effective overall, for all of us. An issue where a personal choice can affect the overall population. When one does not use them as prescribed, and the reason for prescription, the disease comes back, even stronger and requiring another full prescription course, or an even stronger antibiotic, that serves no one properly. Not yourself, not humanity at large.

On Self-Medicating

A few things I'd like to point out here. One should not and I do not, seek medicines/drugs on my own just to make me feel normal, then hang onto that medicine for dear life, blindly continuing to take it. Sure, that was my aim and goal in a way. But I also had to realize...I'm using myself as test subject.

I would not start taking something and if it worked, just keep taking it forever. That can lead to delusional long term abuse. I also stop taking it (if and when appropriate) to prove the case in testing they're actually working. My goal always is to get off of drugs/meds as soon as possible. Then I can see if that's indeed what's making me feel better.

The goal in life as always is to eat naturally in order to be healthy. To live long and get to a point and then remain at optimal/nominal performance and health. And to do that all without the use of drugs, supplements, or unnecessary procedures.

Sure, it's good those things exist, to help us to be normal. But "optimal" would actually be eating food as medicine and using as natural a substance as possible (i.e., herbs, etc.), over harsher chemicals and semi-synthetics. I think of examples of those who are taking handfuls of supplements daily and I just don't see how that is "healthy".

Regarding Testing/Experimenting On Yourself

Beware pop medical claims, charlatans, and "snake oil" salesman. Do take the considered and informed risk that your trusted doctor isn't one of those. As in life and as I've said, as you go, trust, but verify. If you don't have expertise, which most of us don't, find someone you can trust who does. Verified preferably over time, in practice and by word of mouth from trusted friends and loved ones.

Just not some fool on the internet in merely assuming they "might" be good. Or others online in their cohort who only think they're good. It takes more than that. That's how we ended up with people doing bizarre things to damage or kill themselves (and others in their spreading more bad info), in order to "cure" themselves of COVID-19.

Politically speaking, avoid supporting (or voting) for people who are liars, grifters, or seeking power for power's sake. All while convincing their supporters how it's all about them and not those supporters. When in reality they'll make sure they will come well before their supporters or clients (or the country).

I only mention this because we have indeed seen some bad politicians, bad media personalities, bad religious types. Even bad medical professionals (some real, some not), who grifted the public with fake medical cures. Medicine is not politics. It's science. So be aware, and beware. There's nothing lower than abusing those with a delicate constitutions for their own personal gain, at the expense of those they claim to be "helping".

Especially beware those naturally trusted "religious" leaders. Like "ex-con" and current "conman", Jim Bakker. Or any others of his type and hype who try to sell cures for conditions they have no business being involved in. Especially, in using religion to bizarrely support their even more bizarre beliefs of medical (or, other) "cures".

For myself, I've always been logically and scientifically based. A university trained individual who, I grant you, never got a state license to practice therapy. Though the head of our university therapy department did try rather hard to convince me to switch divisions (from "awareness and reasoning"). In his opinion, he thought I'd make a very good therapist.

I was flattered. But my goal is what it always had been at that time, research and writing. That education and training had sharpened my critical skills. Which I always seemed to have a natural inclination toward and if you could ask my parents, they would agree. Even going back to when I was a young kid.

I've had jobs where people's lives depended on my decisions. Though that doesn't carry a lot of weight nowadays. We've seen too many people anymore in very high-end jobs, who act far too inappropriately. Those who should be very responsible people, who should be very good critical thinkers, whose decisions many lives depend on, but who got into business or politics and then went right off the deep end. Something their younger selves might ask of them: "Whatever the hell happened to you [me]?"

Not to worry. This isn't really that hard to maneuver. Just use common sense and...verify, verify, verify.

Diet

I'm not going to preach any particular diet. My normal diet has basically been, healthy. Certainly after my younger years of little or no money, especially while in college. I cut out sugar years ago. Though I still have some sweets from time to time. I do not eat corn syrup at all anymore. I've long tried to live with the orientation of variety, and moderation in all things. Variety, especially in diet.

As for moderation, I found Asian philosophies rather reasonable in their way of thinking. Something I picked up in my readings and as a kid in Karate. But also because of a retired special forces neighbor turned counselor. I asked him one day what his one best piece of advice would be to me.

I was in my early 20s and in the USAF but living in a neighborhood downtown. The south hill of Spokane, Washington. It's a beautiful and rather well off area. He was counseling vets with mental health issues and I thought he was a good and reasonable person to ask something like this. He thought for a moment, then just said, "Moderation." Then he headed out on his morning run, and I headed to the air base.

A modest and varied diet is pretty healthy. Eating the same diet for years, may not give us all we need. Varying our diet, in a health way, offers an easy way to get a variety of the healthy ingredients we need to live on. A nutritionist told me that decades ago and I thought it a great piece of advice.

Also, we eat well most of the time so that once in a while we can indulge and have a little fun. I had a friend at work who years ago would say that corn syrup was "Satan". I'd laugh him off in a friendly way, but he'd say, "Look, I'm serious." Over time I started to pay attention to him on that. Was he onto something? I didn't buy the "Satan" comment, but he also didn't literally mean it, just metaphorically Research and practice however showed he was correct. I started to cut it out of my diet. Easier said than done. It seemed to be in everything.

I finally tested it out one day by eating cookies made with corn syrup. Which also has various names (inverted sugar, glucose syrup, maize syrup, glucose syrup, fruit fructose, crystalline fructose, etc.), making it even harder to eliminate.

I found for me, that compared to cookies made with sugar (or no sugar), the corn syrup cookies always ended me up with eating the entire box over the course of an evening. I just didn't want to stop. Conversely however, with cookies made with sugar I could stop eating them without issue. That was enough proof. So, I tried harder to cut all corn syrup from my life. That's when I realized just how prevalent it is.

I monitor my meat and protein intake, too. I'm an omnivore, not a vegetarian (though I was while in the USAF), but hI aven't eaten much red meat per week in years. Though I love a good steak, I only have one a month or so, no more ever than one a week. It's good to note that many older people do not get enough protein. Too little, or too much, are both health issues. I found research about that some years ago and started paying attention. Too much, turns to fat.

Too little and you can have health issues. I noticed recently when I had to go to a "wound clinic" for an ankle accident I had and a wound that got infected. They may it clear to eat a little more protein daily that I usually did, just until the wound was "sealed and healed".

My annual physicals and blood tests have always been good. Even very good, except for cholesterol, for which I take the "statin". My brother also has that problem. So it seems to be a family trait, which my doctor pointed out. Though my younger half-brother and I didn't grow up together, we're good friends who reconnected as adults. That was decades back now, when our dad died. After my teens, I only saw my dad again a few times. I was pretty young when he had my brother, along with the nine other kids he had married into. So, I guess I understand his disinterest, in a way. Though according to my brother, they all knew all of my accomplishments all through my life.

So after contracting my last version of LC, I felt suddenly hypersensitive to (seemingly) all food. If not actually allergic to whatever I ate. I quickly became afraid of eating. That first week I ate mostly hard boiled eggs.

I tried just one egg that first day, when I realized I seemed to be having pulse and blood pressure spikes to eating, or soon after. Some foods didn't affect me much until they hit my small intestine. I carefully added nuts on the second day. I always keep Costco mixed nuts around. I tried each type of nut separately first, until I realized they were all fine.

That first week after my last infection on March 29th, 2022, where I was dealing with paramedics and the ED visit, I basically just ate those hard boiled eggs, nuts and frozen broccoli florets that I keep around. I typically have some fresh fruits and vegetables, but I keep a backstock of frozen veggies. Frozen veggies have been proven to be as healthy as fresh, and more so than canned. Though fresh is best, it doesn't much matter, as long as you get them.

I lost ten pounds that first week. That I must say, I was all for. I had finally gotten out of the 220lb range and down into the 210s. I've also been 6'2" most of my life (down to 6'1" now in my old age). I'd been trying for years to get the weight down so...the "LC diet"? OK. Sadly perhaps, these symptoms made that diet vastly undesirable.

Hope

We are making ongoing medical advances regarding SARS (Severe Acute Respiratory Syndrome) in general, and in COVID-19, specifically. We continue to learn more every day. A recent discovery in one of those (see, ref# 6) claimed: "Scientific Breakthrough Against COVID-19: Antibodies Identified That May Make Coronavirus Vaccines Unnecessary":

> "Tel Aviv University scientists have isolated two antibodies that neutralize all known strains of COVID-19 – including Omicron – with up to 95% efficiency."

Well, that would be nice. There will be many more (and already some) advances. I've included some of that information throughout this book and in the ending reference section. But our biggest hope is in ourselves.

Look, listen, and whenever we can research on our own. Even consider joining research studies as subjects. Those things alone can help us a great deal overall and even motivate us. Learning as we can, whenever we can, along our path out of this LC medical mess helps to distract one, if nothing else.

I remember thinking when I first got sick with COVID, that I should keep a log. But I was so disabled, so lacking in energy, I quickly gave it up as wishful thinking. I remember considering writing a book about my experiences as I was living through it. But I quickly and frustratingly realized that was simply impossible. It was depressing.

My log keeping should actually have been far better than it turned out as I knew what I was capable of. But that would have required a much better mindset, and so much more energy, and much more clarity of mind and even, outright desire than I could muster. Certainly, in the beginning during that first year long bout of LC.

Or maybe, I just needed help. But there was only myself, here. From time to time a family member would come by. But they all live in other towns. Those visits did help though. Just in someone being there, even for a short visit, helps.

However, we had lock downs, fears of infecting another, especially our loved ones. It was a difficult time all around and for everyone. I'm just thankful I did not go through some of the horrors many others did, regarding their family and loved ones. My heart deeply goes out to them. And there's been so very many of them.

COVID, is a miserable disease in far too many ways. There will surely be more of this in the future. What might a COVID-30 bring if we don't quickly get a handle on it overall? Though we have made some great strides already.

Still, we also have to get a better grasp on how we live in general. And in how we produce and process our foods. How we destructively encroach on wilderness. How we abuse and concentrate ourselves beyond reasonable limits for our environments. And merely in our typical living conditions.

Remember at all some time ago people said, "small is beautiful"? That was also from a 1973 book, "Small Is Beautiful: Economics as if People Mattered", by EF Schumacher. Best known for his proposals for human-scale, decentralized and appropriate technologies. That title alone was great advice from the head economist of India decades ago. (see his quotes, ref# 24)

Schumacher suggested localized energy generation. As we're now starting to do with solar panels. Though they took a while to become cost effective and available for consumers, they were invented in 1954. They were made available to the pubic in the late 1970s. Jimmy Carter installed them on the White House in 1979. Then bizarrely, Pres. Reagan removed them. Politics over reality, again.

I first read Schumacher's rather charming book while vacationing in Hawaii, in 1978. I was quite taken with it. I mention it because we do need to look at small fixes, and at ourselves sometimes. Over the typically big "fixes" that tend to be so bad as long term fixes.

I got my updated COVID booster, on Monday, September 12, 2022. So I'll end this section here, with that updated booster. I still have LC. It may go on for months longer [Note: I'm revising this book and today is January 2, 2024; I still have (20 months in so far now) it but it's lighter than ever and only flares up a bit here and there]. Though hopefully no longer than that. But I have to end this somewhere, just so I can get this book out for others to see.

Maybe the next shot I get will be the last [it now appears to be an annual shot like flu, for now], in it being a new type of medicine. I hope it is and soon, with no more vaccines or boosters needed. One can only hope that a new medicine will end SARS in general, and not just COVID-19. Along with LC, as well.

I spent nearly a year unable to do much at all. Striving to have some degree of motivation or energy. To even be motivated at all. But I never gave up. Nearly perhaps, a few times. But then, as I felt myself feeling more energetic (an overstatement), or perhaps just as I got used to my condition enough to work through it (most likely a bit of both), I continued to push myself, but carefully.

Always trying to do at least a bit more than before. I would be\ perfectly happy if I could only get to a point where I don't notice LC anymore. When it could then take it's sweet time finally to burn completely out. [I'm kind of there now. I did see new research about some finding their vagus nerve had thickened and I hope that's not me but statistically, hopefully not]

Next up as I finish writing this book, I'm finally taking my son's advice and trying cannabis CBD isolate (lacking THC, an oil you put drops of in your mouth.). It helps for issues of inflammation and I'm hoping also, for LC inflammation. Which we're finding has a lot to do with LC. I know at least one person in the online LC group said he couldn't make it, without his CBDs.

Yes, I still have LC. Though it's much better than it had been. I've learned how to make it less noticeable and irritating. I do have to continue exercising, taking Benadryl as needed (less and less anymore), and seeing how CBDs work out for me. Which so far seem to be making my vagus nerve more sensitive not less which is counter intuitive. Which really is just so very LC-like.

Some have said LC burns out within a couple of years. My first go around in 2020 was just over a year. At this moment, this time it's been seven months. It could end any day. Here's hoping. But really, we don't know how long it lasts, yet. Or even why it goes away. But we're learning more every day.

Recently I had an in-home doctor visit from Signify, a benefit of my Aetna supplemental Medicare insurance (though I mostly use VA healthcare). The doctor said I look healthy. BP was 100/over something, good. A bit low, but better than the 140/over something at a dental appointment I had a few days before his visit.

I'm wondering if CBDs had to do with healthier levels of blood pressure, after only two days of use? Less inflammation, less high BP? But I'm also thinking it had to do with the air quality issues being better now.

There's always going to be set backs. Always are. But try not to see a "wall" you can't push through. If you do, never let it stop you. Not until you're, yourself. That's how we win.

With that, I wish you all good health!

Cheers! Na zdravie! Sláinte!

Chapter 7

Update: Long Covid — Evolving Science and Integrated Understanding (2025)

When I first revised this book in early 2024, Long Covid remained poorly defined in both clinical practice and public understanding.

While its reality was no longer disputed, explanations for *why* it persisted, recycled, or manifested so differently from person to person were still fragmented. Research was emerging rapidly, but conclusions were cautious, provisional, and often disconnected.

I would like to return briefly to my first COVID-19 infection, the one that began presenting symptoms in early 2020. I referenced it early in this book, but only recently did I pause long enough to look closely at the numbers from that period. What I discovered put my experience in a very different light.

When my first COVID-19 symptoms appeared on **February 9, 2020**, the United States was still officially recognizing only a very small number of confirmed infections. Retrospective analyses show that, through most of February, the country had documented **fewer than two dozen confirmed cases**, most of them linked directly to international travel. Community transmission would not even be formally acknowledged until later that month.

For most people in America, the moment it became clear that COVID was truly here came on **February 26, 2020**, when the first reported deaths at the Life Care Center in Kirkland were announced. That nursing home, only about twenty-three miles across Puget Sound from where I live, suddenly became the focus of national attention as the first deadly outbreak recognized in the United States. That news broke **fourteen days after** I had already been through the worst of my own illness.

Those official numbers from that time do not reflect the true spread of the virus. Testing was extremely limited, and early surveillance criteria were so narrow that many infections were simply never identified.

Even so, the counts we do have make one thing unmistakably clear. My illness occurred extraordinarily early. I was part of what I think of as the "quiet phase" of the pandemic in this country, when COVID was already moving through communities, but before most people, including much of the medical system, fully realized it was here.

In the week before I became sick, I had only been out in public twice. One outing was to "Slash Night Shorts," a late night, monthly indie film event that my friend and fellow director Kelly Hughes and I founded (short lived due to the pandemic), held at the historic Roxy Theater here in Bremerton, Washington.

The other was a simple trip to a local grocery store. At that point in early 2020, the known incubation period for COVID-19 was generally understood to be between two and fourteen days, with most people developing symptoms about five to six days after exposure.

Looking back with that knowledge, either of those outings could easily have been the moment I encountered the virus, especially the film event, which gathered filmmakers and fans from across Kitsap county in close proximity, at a time when none of us yet realized the virus was already circulating.

Realizing now just how early my illness occurred gives new context to everything that followed. With that perspective in mind, it becomes even more important to look at where things stand today, and what has changed since those first quiet, unseen days of the pandemic.

That is what finally struck me the other day. I had been sick weeks before America even understood the virus was here. Weeks before the "first deaths." Weeks before the headlines. I was already fighting COVID while the nation still slept, part of that first silent wave that moved through the country unnoticed, unrecognized, and utterly unprepared.

By 2025, the quiet fear of those early days had become something else entirely. The world knew the virus now. What it was still struggling to understand was everything it left behind.

There is still no single cause, no universal treatment, and no clean resolution for all who suffer from Long Covid. What has changed, however, is that multiple independent lines of research are now converging on a **coherent explanatory framework** (see, ref #68, #71, #77). This framework does not simplify Long Covid, but it does make it more comprehensible.

This chapter replaces the earlier 2024 update and reflects the most current understanding as of 2025, integrating institutional research with the lived experience detailed throughout this book.

Long Covid as a Syndrome, Not a Single Disease

One of the most important developments since 2024 is the growing consensus that Long Covid is **not a single post-viral condition**, but a **syndrome composed of overlapping biological mechanisms** (see, ref #68, #69, #77).

Long Covid is now commonly understood to involve varying combinations of:

1. Persistent immune dysregulation

2. Reactivation of latent viruses

3. Residual inflammatory triggers or viral antigens

4. Autonomic and metabolic disruption

Not every patient experiences all of these, and no two cases present identically. This helps explain why standardized treatment approaches often fail and why symptom patterns can shift over time (see, ref #77).

This is why the condition can make sufferers feel, at times, as though they are losing their minds—why so much of it seems to have no rationale or logic. It is not you. It is the disease.

Viral Reactivation: From Hypothesis to Substantial Evidence

By 2025, the reactivation of latent viruses—particularly **Epstein-Barr virus (EBV)** and other **herpes-family viruses (HSV)**—is no longer considered a fringe hypothesis (see, ref #29, #71).

Multiple studies now show that a meaningful subset of Long Covid patients demonstrate immune markers consistent with **recent or ongoing viral reactivation**, including elevated antibody titers and immune dysregulation patterns similar to other post-viral syndromes (see, ref #29). Antibody titers are a quantitative measure of antibodies in the blood—specifically, how much of a particular antibody (for example, against SARS-CoV-2) is present.

Importantly, this does not imply that SARS-CoV-2 itself becomes a chronic infection in most patients. Rather, COVID-19 appears unusually effective at **disrupting immune surveillance**, allowing dormant viruses—sometimes held in check for decades—to re-emerge (see, ref #71, #77).

This framework helps explain:

- symptom flares without reinfection

- delayed onset following apparent recovery

- partial response to antiviral strategies

- cycling or relapsing symptom patterns

Immune and Hormonal Dysregulation

Another area of increasing clarity involves **immune-hormonal imbalance**, particularly disruptions involving cortisol regulation and inflammatory signaling (see, ref #71, #77).

Research now supports that some Long Covid patients exhibit **lower-than-expected cortisol levels**, alongside persistent immune activation and abnormal T-cell signaling (see, ref #71). This does not necessarily indicate adrenal failure, but rather dysfunction in the normal feedback loops that regulate inflammation and stress response.

Clinically, this may manifest as:

- fatigue disproportionate to exertion

- post-exertional malaise

- exaggerated stress responses

- impaired recovery following physical or cognitive effort

These findings align closely with symptom clusters identified in NIH-funded cohort studies (see, ref #77, #82).

Persistent Antigens and Chronic Inflammation

Separate from viral reactivation, research has identified **persistent SARS-CoV-2 antigens**, including spike protein fragments, in certain tissues long after acute infection (see, ref #71, #78).

While this does not necessarily indicate active viral replication, persistent antigens may be sufficient to:

- maintain low-grade immune activation

- disrupt endothelial and vascular function

- perpetuate inflammatory signaling

This mechanism may coexist with viral reactivation rather than replace it, suggesting that Long Covid may involve **both ongoing immune provocation and secondary viral consequences** (see, ref #71, #77).

This, in particular, caused significant difficulty for me early on, especially in 2023, when I was trying to explain to my VA physician what I was experiencing. I repeatedly described symptoms that, by 2023–2024, increasingly appeared to reflect Long Covid acting as a trigger for another condition rather than as a single, self-contained illness.

The medication I was requesting—Valacyclovir for HSV—was repeatedly dismissed on the grounds that it does not treat Long Covid, which is true. But as I tried to explain, it *was* helping me. Not by treating Long Covid itself, as I eventually came to understand in listening to my doctor, but as I learned through research, by suppressing HSV reactivation that appeared to have been triggered by the Long Covid–related immune disruption.

It took considerable time before I was finally prescribed a maintenance dose of Valacyclovir—500 mg daily. In my own review of clinical literature and physician reports, I found that higher doses, including 1,000 mg daily, had historically been used in some cases to manage persistent HSV activity. At that dosage —either as a single 1,000 mg dose or split into two 500 mg doses —I experienced a near-complete absence of HSV-related symptoms.

Despite this, I was unable to persuade my physician to adopt that dosing strategy beyond short-term flare management. Mostly because it was a VA rule, going against what was being done around the world elsewhere.

Eventually, he agreed that I could use 1,000 mg daily during flare-ups in addition to the maintenance dose. Much of my success in convincing him had to do with my monitoring, documenting and sharing that information with him. And it took time, frustrating (and painful) as that was.

I want to stress that throughout this experience I had made up my mind to make a consistent effort to trust my physician while also verifying what I was experiencing through careful observation, research, and follow-up reporting.

I believe in the end that he was correct in dosage and prescription. When I was told this may be my prescription for life, I could not accept it. I refused to accept it. I was already on statins for my cholesterol issues, prevalent in my family. They take a toll on your liver. Adding Valacyclovir to that adds additional burden, albeit in a different fashion.

With statins the advisement is to limit oneself to one or two alcoholic beverages a day. Adding Valacyclovir, adds an additional warning. I'm not a big drinker, but it is a gauge by which I've judged my long Covid-ness. Sugar and alcohol indicate how I'm doing. There was a time during Long Covid, when having a drink, or eating sugar, made me feel like I was going to die.

To me, that additional medication was a burden on my liver I did not want to live with. So I dug into research and tried various things to get off the Valacyclovir.

Eventually I found that lysine has long been used for HSV issues and I tried it. I wish I had known that as a kid when I had a painful cold sore. And so, I got off the Valacyclovir. The next obvious step is to get off the lysine, although it's far less of concern than the medication. L-lysine is one of the nine **essential amino acids**, meaning the human body cannot synthesize it and must obtain it from diet or supplementation.

- **Valacyclovir** is a **prodrug** of acyclovir, meaning it is converted by the body into the active antiviral compound acyclovir.

- It works by **inhibiting viral DNA replication**, specifically against herpesviruses such as HSV-1, HSV-2, and varicella-zoster.

For HSV, lysine acts upstream of antiviral drugs by **altering the biochemical environment the virus depends on**, rather than directly blocking viral DNA replication.

I would prefer to prevent, rather than suppress.

Looking back, I recognize that I provided my physician with far more information than was practical within the constraints of routine clinical care. I made a conscious effort to be circumspect, fully aware that he was a busy physician managing many complex cases. Still, I felt strongly that what I was uncovering might be relevant beyond my own situation and could ultimately benefit other veterans as well.

But the system just doesn't seem to be set up that way.

At one point, he explained—politely and candidly in a VA email —that while he found the material interesting, he was responsible for a large number of patients, some of whom were in extremely poor condition due to serious service-related injuries.

In that context, he noted that I was, comparatively speaking, one of his healthiest patients, Long Covid notwithstanding. He also emphasized that he was not a research physician, nor was the massive Puget Sound Veterans Health Care System facility, a research facility.

I understood his position, but it was nonetheless disheartening. What I needed at that stage was not only clinical care, but investigation. At the time I was seeking answers, the VA did not yet have a visible or accessible Long Covid research component integrated into everyday clinical practice at my facility.

Although national VA research initiatives have since been developed, those efforts were not available at the point of care during the early years of my illness. I had after all, contracted COVID-19 and Long Covid early in February 2020 when few new what was going on. As a result, many veterans—including myself—were left navigating Long Covid largely on our own, without a coordinated research or response framework embedded in clinical settings.

I was fortunate in that I had formal university training and a career in the IT industry that required rigorous research skills. Applying those skills to medical and pharmacological literature was not a significant leap, as I had drawn on them in earlier decades out of both professional necessity, and out of personal curiosity in the realms of medicine and scientific research.

I note this because frustration can lead some patients to ignore or dismiss their physicians altogether. If you do not trust your doctor, the appropriate response is to seek another—not to disregard medical training and clinical experience, which can be dangerous. Or with this disease, disastrous.

What ultimately proved necessary in my case was a collaborative approach: educating myself while working with a physician willing to listen, and maintaining mutual respect rather than dismissal on either side. And the hardest part was accepting that this process required time.

I took the prescribed medication during a period when it significantly reduced pain and distress—something that, at the time, felt lifesaving. Eventually, however, I found that I could achieve comparable, and in some respects better, stability not by continually suppressing viral activity pharmacologically, but by reducing the likelihood of viral reactivation in the first place through the use of lysine (500 mg daily, with 1,000 mg used briefly—two to three days, up to five—during flare ups).

My physician is fully aware of this approach, which I continue with his knowledge and advisement.

Autonomic Nervous System Involvement

Growing attention has also been paid to the **autonomic nervous system**, including vagus nerve signaling (see, ref #73, #74, #77). I learned a lot about the vagus nerve in this process, as I've previously noted.

Some Long Covid patients experience dysautonomia-like symptoms such as heart rate variability issues, blood pressure instability, gastrointestinal disturbance, and heightened sensitivity to stress. In most cases, this appears to reflect **functional dysregulation rather than structural nerve damage**, likely driven by persistent immune and inflammatory signaling.

This reinforces the understanding that Long Covid involves cross-system interactions between immune, neurological, and metabolic pathways rather than a single organ-specific pathology.

Where Lysine Fits — Carefully and Contextually

As research increasingly supports viral reactivation as a contributing mechanism in Long Covid, it becomes appropriate to revisit one aspect of my own experience: **lysine supplementation**.

Lysine is not a treatment for COVID-19 or Long Covid. It is not a cure. Nor should it be assumed safe or appropriate for all individuals.

However, lysine has a long-documented role as an **adjunct in suppressing replication of certain herpes-family viruses**, particularly through interactions with arginine metabolism (see, ref #85). Its relevance lies not in treating Long Covid directly, but in **modulating secondary viral activity** under conditions of immune stress.

In my case, lysine correlated with:

- reduced symptom flares

- greater stability over time

- fewer episodes consistent with viral reactivation

This does not establish causation nor generalize broadly. Within the 2025 framework—where viral reactivation is no longer speculative—it offers a **mechanistically coherent explanation** for why it may have been beneficial *for me*.

I include this not as guidance, but as illustration.

This is something I just learned about the other day. Lysine and arginine are competing amino acids, and this distinction matters for herpesvirus reactivation. HSV relies on arginine to replicate, while lysine competes with arginine for absorption and cellular use.

By shifting that balance, lysine does not treat Long Covid directly, nor does it eradicate HSV, but it can reduce the likelihood of viral reactivation in susceptible individuals. In my case, this distinction proved crucial.

Why Recovery Is Often Slow and Non-Linear

The emerging 2025 model suggests that recovery from Long Covid occurs not when a virus disappears, but when **regulatory balance is restored** (see, ref #77).

This may involve:

- recalibration of immune signaling

- suppression of latent viral activity

- normalization of hormonal feedback loops

- gradual stabilization of autonomic function

This process is slow, uneven, and often incomplete. Understanding this does not eliminate suffering, but it replaces confusion with context.

Closing Perspective

As of 2025, Long Covid remains complex—but it is no longer inexplicable.

The distance between patient experience and scientific explanation is narrowing (see, ref #68, #71, #77). The science is increasingly reflecting what patients have long reported: that Long Covid is real, biologically grounded, and multifactorial.

This update represents the most integrated understanding available as I could find it. It does not erase earlier uncertainty—just explains it.

As throughout this book, this chapter reflects my experience interpreted through evolving science, not medical advice, prescription, or universal claims.

Chapter 8

My Daily Long Covid Logs

2020/2021

As previously mentioned, I first caught COVID-19 the first time, that is first showing symptoms on Sunday, February 9, 2020. I was so out of it for most of that year, that it didn't initially occur to me to keep a daily log. Though I had considered writing a book about it, as I've said. But a daily log only came up when I realized that no doctor I was seeing, had very much info on Long Covid. I needed some "weight", some proof behind my words. It proved highly effective in sharing parts of this log with my doctor.

I needed documentation to prove my contentions to doctors who thought I was incorrect. Or, mad? Or just delusional? Luckily I didn't run into that, exactly. But there was difficultly in them acting more proactively on what I was saying. To be fair, in part because because they still had so little information themselves and in the beginning none at all.

So I began maintaining a log and started saving research I came across for medical personal. But as they pointed out, they're not a research facility. Which struck me as odd. Albeit, it was honest and realistic of them to say. Which was too also bad (for me, and others), as I felt, shouldn't every medical facility at least to some degree, be a research facility? It begged the question for me:

"Where were the Long Covid specialist teams for those of us with LC?"

Especially at the Veterans Administration. I had over eight months of LC after I got over my initial 2020 infection. It took several months for my lungs to return to reasonable health, and nearly an entire year before they began to feel normal again. I considered they may never return to normal.

There was a long bout of lethargy, or malaise. A general feeling of bodily discomfort, fatigue or unpleasantness at the onset of COVID, which continued on for the rest of that year and into the next. I tired easily, had marked "brain fog", and forgetfulness. I became concerned that I may never again be able to write a book. Or even a short story. I kept finding noticeable events of forgetfulness that were ever more disturbing. But luckily, thankfully, that has all passed.

For most of 2020 and winter going into 2021, I was in my living room recliner watching TV, or on my laptop. Or drifting into sleep. It was difficult to concentrate for long on anything. I would drift off to sleep while watching, mostly "binging", on some TV series or other. Which seemed a better fit for my condition. They became my go to as I was spending such long periods glued to my TV. "Glued" was relative, as viewing was such a tenuous thing.

I noticed more recently, having forgotten I had watched some film or TV series in 2020, that I would remember having watched it, after starting to watch it again (not realizing at first that I was re-watching it). I would come to realize I had indeed seen the show before. It was a strange experience.

Until finally one day I realized that must have been what was going on. Because I had previously been watching while going in and out of consciousness. It took me a few different shows until I made that realization. Which pointedly showed me what a very strange existence I'd had that first year of LC.

Oddly, as I came out of LC in 2021, I noticed my memory actually seemed better in ways it hadn't been, prior to COVID's onset. As if it had cleared memory pathways. Or more likely, rebuilt some of those pathways. I found I seemed to have better pathways than before. I was remembering types of things that in 2019 I'd had more difficulty remembering. It was an odd, but pleasant experience. Disturbing nonetheless, as I'd heard so much in the news about the damage COVID could do. This was actually a more welcome possibility. One I'd never heard anyone mention.

The following is from my personal logs on my two year (and counting) LC experience. I've cleaned it up a little bit for inclusion here, but it's purposely still a bit rough. I left it like that because I believe it better exhibits the depths of some of my condition, my fears and concerns, irritations and frustrations. Also regarding LC, my healthcare and our general lack of knowledge and ability at appropriate handling of those of us suffering from Long Covid.

After initially speaking with my Veterans Administration physician, he had me get an MRI to check for brain damage from COVID-19, and Long Covid.

"Oh, great!' I thought at the time. But then, it really is best to find out, and ASAP!

So here are my logs. I'll begin with the results of that MRI/Brain Scan, on 7/9/21:

CLINICAL HISTORY: Forgetfulness since COVID infection in February 2021. [that should say 2020]

COMPARISON: No relevant comparisons are available at the time of dictation.

TECHNIQUE: MRI of the brain was performed utilizing multiplanar multiecho technique.? Neither intravenous nor intra-articular contrast was administered.

FINDINGS: The brain midline structures are intact. The ventricles and CSF spaces are within normal limits. There is mild bilateral anterior frontal lobe volume loss. No brain midline shift or mass lesion is present. There are nonspecific few small foci of

T2 hyperintensity within bilateral periventricular and superior deep white matter, consistent with microangiopathic ischemic changes. (see, ref# 25)

No evidence for acute infarct or ischemia is present. The sella is within normal limits and no perisellar or suprasellar mass is present. The central major intracranial vessel flow voids are maintained. No abnormal extra-axial fluid collections are present. The orbits are intact. No paranasal sinus opacification is present. And when I say I got up at night to "relieve" myself, I mean, urinate.

2022

1 March 2022

Started feeling a general ill feeling/illness.

10 March 2022

Started taking krill oil as research indicated it was good for the heart. [That lasted for 35 days ending 4/8/22 because in researching it, I made a connection in what it can do to cause issues I was having.]

Two weeks before my youngest son (& spouse) came over (eldest son lives hours away, in Yakima), arriving minutes after my first tachycardia episode (3/10/22). I had been several days on krill oil. Was it just that supplement, or another LC episode prior to my next COVID infection, that occurred on or around 3/28/22 (when symptoms were so grossly exhibited)?

Before they arrived I felt like I might need a hospital. My pulse spiked to 130. I drank water, walked in the yard, calming down. Within a few hours I felt like I'd peaked on an illness, as if something had died in me (like a virus).

11 March 2022 Friday

Feeling like I caught something. Though I may be over it by Saturday. But feeling lethargic, with fast heartbeat, and feeling I'm fighting something off.

Final thought, maybe it IS Long Covid again/still, just recycling. [this kind of confusion was forever frustrating, making it hard to diagnose, so I can feel for medical professionals trying to do it for someone not themselves.]

I started standard Valacyclovir schedule (two pills per day, for three days) because I felt a potential normal herpes flare up coming on. I recently finished a course for a flare up just a couple of weeks before, just before the sickness started which had begun with sinus congestion/pain (as had COVID-19 on Feb. 9th 2020.

13 March 2022 Sunday

Kids came over again. Feel better but now, maybe just a cold.

16 March 2022 Wednesday

Still feel horrible, but not like the past two weeks. I feel "ill" of being ill for so long, I'm so sick of it.

17 March 2022 Thursday

St. Patrick's Day! Feeling better. Had five very tasty pints of Guinness and a couple shots of Jameson over the day, and just fun stuff to eat today. I'm missing hitting an Irish pub on this holiday.

18 March 2022 Friday

Feel a little burnt from the beers, but feeling pretty good. Still feels like a light cold, fading.

22 March 2022 Tuesday

Twenty-one days now. Feeling ever better, having had two too many whiskeys, two days ago. Feeling lung issues slightly still, but continuing to get over this thing.

24 March 2022 Thursday

Still not well, maybe it's partially seasonal allergies. Did not take nightly atorvastatin [for cholesterol] last night in case that's part of the issue.

28 March 2022 Sunday

Omicron Variant COVID-19 infection symptoms began [with a nod to the previous experience, not really knowing where to place that in explaining what happened here overall].

[And the nightmare begins...]

I felt weird. Took Benadryl at 10PM after son & spouse left.

At bed time took 81mg aspirin (doctor had me on that for the past year, but when the government came out saying not to take it unless you have a specific reason, I had stopped it and take it now only for blood clot issues from COVID).

I had a tachycardia (medical term for heart rate over 100 beats a minute) episode requiring a call to 911. Paramedics arrived 2:30AM. [I drove myself a few hours later to ER at St. Michael's Medical Center, Emergency Department in Silverdale, WA, eleven miles from home.]

29 March 2022 Monday

2AM Woke with high blood pressure & pulse up to and sustained at 140beats per minutes. So, tachycardia and for no apparent reason.

BP 157/89, but it had gone down by then, this about 20 minutes after I got up. Could not get heart rate down and so I called 911. Paramedics came and I was feeling better by then and my stats looked better.

They suggested a trip to the ED, ASAP. I said I could drive myself. They agreed that may be correct.

I left west Bremerton on the two mile drive to Harrison Medical Center and got lost in east Bremerton. I had used this hospital for nearly two decades and it's odd not easily finding. After a near panic attack, frustration and exhaustion, I finally found it after about 30 minutes. [I later discovered it had been closed for 6 months.]

By then I felt better, so I drove home, got my pulse down to 88 and decided to try to sleep.

I woke too soon. about 6AM. I got up, exhausted. I realized after a bit that my heart rate was back up and had gone to 140. I called the VA help line and talked to someone who transferred me to the nurse who said, yes, I should go to the ED. I told her about the event last night and she assured me again that yes, go to St. Michael's ED in Silverdale.

I drove to St. Michael's ED a little after 8AM. I did not feel well driving there and was hoping I could make it, not knowing what was going on with me.

Forty minutes in the ED waiting area after checking in, I was taken to an ED ward room. They hooked me up to monitors and everything looked good. They drew blood and the blood tests came back looking good. I asked for a COVID test and they denied me that, saying it wouldn't prove anything at that point. I found that confusing, but they were the experts.

They gave me a two week Zio chest patch/heart monitor to wear and a diary card to keep for any unusual incidences. I later downloaded the phone app. To use the monitor, you pushed a button on the patch if you experienced an event. Then later, you could fill in what you were experiencing in the app on your phone. This was handy for events that wake you in the middle of the night.

I felt better, but tired from lack of sleep and four hours in the ED lying on one of those small medical work beds. I drove home. At home my pulse was, 97.

I called the VA to update them about the 911 & ED visits, mostly for administrative and financial reasons.

After all this I realized I had forgotten to mention I'd been using Fluticasone Propionate Glucocorticoid steroid sinus spray (suggested by my doctor, a while back). I stopped using that immediately.

St. Michael Medical Center - Silverdale: Emergency Room

1800 Northwest Myhre Road First Floor, Silverdale, WA 98383 - 360 744-8800

Notify VA about ED visit within 72 hours

Called VA for approval 844 724-7842 - 3/28/22 12:41pm

Saved notification ID# they supplied me with on the phone.

30 April 2022 Saturday

The previous period from ED visit to today was OK but my pulse seemed at times unnervingly untethered to my physical actions. Something changed with all that today.

Blood Pressure:

I woke with headache and felt I needed to check blood pressure.

First time that happened, ever. The experience of having such high blood pressure for the first time, after weeks of my pulse being an issue, was further anxiety evoking.

6:16AM 168 / 88

6:19AM 160 / 90

6:23AM 159 / 92

6:24AM 164 / 91

6:27AM 161 / 93

Called 911

Monitored with 911 Operator as I waited for Paramedics:

181 / 101 [note that here I did not indicate time, as it was hard to think clearly]

6:38AM 145 85

6:40AM 144 / 86

6:52AM 132 / 86

Bedtime, at this point I started taking BP upon rising and at bedtime, at VA Nurse's suggestion for the next time I spoke to my doctor:

10:53PM 131 / 77 pulse 79

1 May 2022 Sunday

Morning

5:35AM 140 / 78 pulse 83

5:39AM 120 / 75 pulse 75

Bedtime:

10:20PM 132 / 76 pulse 85

2 May 2022 Monday

Morning

4:47AM 138 / 81 pulse 77

4:48AM 124 / 72 pulse 72

Bedtime:

11PM 128 / 67 pulse 71

3 May 2022 Tuesday

Morning

7:30AM 125 / 69 pulse 80

7:31AM 120 / 68 pulse 74

9:30PM Bedtime: drank Chamomile – great idea, until we wake up to relieve yourself

10:37PM 112 / 64 pulse 64

4 May 2022 Wednesday

Morning

7:05AM 111 / 68 pulse 70

Felt like I was dying this morning. Or maybe just low blood pressure, or something? Overwhelming, overall feeling of BAD. Pulse went up to at least 129 for a while. BP was not bad.

11AM Finally, took a 500mg Valacyclovir and almost immediately felt better. Expected it to fail, but hoped it would work. Thought it was placebo effect at first, but starting to think this isn't catching a new virus, but a re-occurrence [reactivation] of herpes virus with no specific areas of pain or visible phenomena, just overall disturbing illness.

By 12:20PM as I was eating lunch, I was feeling almost normal.

2PM, started to feel the ill feeling again, but not so bad as earlier. Felt like taking another pill sooner than 12 hours, but held off for normal time. Looked it up and found (see above: Varicella-zoster virus reactivation):

"Treatment with Valacyclovir 1000 mg × 3/ day for 7–14 days was efficient in all cases."
3PM feeling better now

5PM took another Valacyclovir

Bedtime:

11:38PM 116 / 69 p 70

Took another Valacyclovir

5 May 2022 Thursday

6AM Took Valacyclovir

Morning, woke feeling more rested but burned out, but not like I'm dying, anyway.

7:18AM 126 / 70 p85

Valacyclovir by 9AM, didn't seem as effective as yesterday

6PM Valacyclovir

Bedtime:

10:30PM 116 / 67 p75

6 May 2022 Friday

6:30AM Valacyclovir

6:30AM 118 / 72 p72

11:18AM Initially 163 / something

11:19AM blood pressure spiked seemingly for no reason

11:19AM 152 / 84 p 91

11:20AM 148 / 81 p78

11:22AM 133 / 82 p74

11:23AM 126 / 80 p72

Bedtime:

11PM Valacyclovir (took 3 today, works better than 2)

7 May 2022 Saturday

7AM Valacyclovir

7:37AM 129 / 76 pulse97

7:38AM 131 / 74 p96

7:40AM 143 / 80 p96

7:42AM 148 / 80 p99

7:43AM 132 / 79 p99

7:46AM 151 / 84 p98

7:46AM 152 / 89 p108

7:53AM 134 / 78 p 96

7:55AM 128 / 79 p86

3PM Valacyclovir

Bedtime:

10:54PM 112 / 66 p73 Valacyclovir

The previous were brought together from various notes I had haphazardly thrown together.

The following is the log I began on May 8th, 2022 and was incidental for me just to keep it all straight in my head. I didn't know I was actually going to keep a legitimate daily log until Tuesday, May 17, 2022.

Which was when it really started to become more than just a personal log for me alone. I kept adding to it up until today, as I write this. While I was keeping this log file updated, as you can see from the previous above, I was also adding files with other information and have moved most of those references and URL links at the end.

8 May 2022 Sunday

Woke with headache, pulsing, feeling a high BP.

Got up, dressed, brushed teeth, sat down, relaxed my muscles/body and began to feel my BP lowering. Waited a few minutes and then took BP.

Stopped taking Valacyclovir Sunday morning (last of a series) 5/8/22 because I was feeling better.

Thought I'd take another at 3PM or 6PM if I felt I needed one.

5:21AM 135 / 76 p80

5:22AM 120 / 79 p75

Bedtime:

11PM 128 / 74 p80

9 May 2022 Monday

Woke feeling pretty good

8:25AM 117 / 71 p72

By noon starting feeling a bit lethargic again.

Felt better about Bedtime:

118 / 69 p68

Final

10 May 2022 Tuesday

7:47AM 113 / 72 p75

Kept waking up as usual lately, but felt pretty good when waking.

Saw VA Doctor. By that night, started feeling it all come back.

[Up to this point my daily logs were used just to track things for myself to note changes. Then I started doing it for my doctor. Eventually, I was keeping the log for a permanent record, or in case I dropped dead. I felt my adult kids would find it and it may be of some use to them. My oldest son lives three hours away in Yakima, WA. While my youngest is in Chimacum, WA, about 50 minutes away.]

4:50PM 130/75 BP

11 May 2022 Wednesday

Woke feeling foggy again and took a Valacyclovir.

Two weeks have gone by, I very happily removed my heart monitor patch and mailed the damn thing in. A patch on your skin for two weeks where you can't clean your skin under it, was to say the least, uncomfortable. Itching, like having a cast on a broken arm. Feeling pretty good today after that, though.

Feeling pretty good today

3PM Took another Valacyclovir.

11PM Another Valacyclovir.

12 May 2022 Thursday

Woke feeling I needed to continue. Three pills today

13 May 2022 Friday

Woke feeling good and wasn't going to take a Valacyclovir.

10AM I started feeling bad again, slightly, but obvious that it was coming back on, so I took another Valacyclovir.

14 May 2022 Saturday

I couldn't sleep until about 2AM.

3AM Woke with bad tachycardia. Did some breathing exercises the VA Nurse gave me. I got up and drank cold water, splashed cold water on my face (and other techniques to lower pulse). I got back to sleep, about three hours of sleep (maybe four) total. I tried to sleep more, but couldn't, so I just got up. So this is my life now...

15 May 2022

email to my VA doctor:

Dr...
I received your messages today via phone call. Thank you. I would like to stop the Valacyclovir, but when I do, I get ill to the point of inability to do anything but sit and be ill. I worry that stopping will bring back my tachycardia and blood pressure issues which still occur, but slightly, infrequently.
I had BP issues start today, took half of a Benadryl and it faded, which is curious. [this I later learned was due to histamine issues, not as my doctor surmised, to the calming effect Benadryl can have]
Here is the email I was writing to you today, before our phone calls:
In trying the past few weeks to use Valacyclovir to feel better, hoping it deactivates the virus so I can stop taking them, I've found a 500mg Valacyclovir 3 times a day fends off the virus. Also, Benadryl has helped get me through this past week, not sure if that's just seasonal allergies or not. It's relieved pressure overall, which doesn't quite seem like normal allergies.

I've tried to get it down to one a day but it's very uncomfortable.
Two is also not great, but 3 (500mg) seems to keep it at bay day & night.
So I'm wondering if maybe two, 1000mg pills a day, would work better?
I would like to get to a point where I can stop taking it, but that doesn't seem to be working. When I stop taking them, my quality of life goes down and all I feel capable of doing is sitting and watching TV, day and night. I woke the other night with tachycardia and only got three hours sleep. I was exhausted and ill all day, but the next time, I slept pretty well. I try to go for walks but so far my blood pressure is problematic, even when taking it easy. I'll keep at it. I feel I just need to get to a certain point and my body will be more functional again.
I had some Valacyclovir left over when I recently accidentally ordered two prescriptions at once. Thinking one didn't go through on the website, I contacted your office. But I'm now almost out.
Can I get more ASAP before I run out? I have a few left.
When they wear off, it becomes very uncomfortable. I get a bit foggy and feel like I've had too much caffeine, a bit weak and shaky, like my body is fighting hard to fend off an infection.
Thank you."
END EMAIL.

At this point I went back and forth with the nurse who was adamant the doctor would not give me Valacyclovir for other than what it was intended for. Talking to him direct was different. I believe this email changed his mind however, and I did get a thirty day supply, for two (not three) pills per day. Throughout all of this going forward, I did my best to follow his orders.

16 May 2022 Monday

Feeling better this morning.

Restarted atorvastatin (cholesterol meds) after speaking with my VA doctor.

Later, I started feeling a bit foggy/lethargic again.

17 May 2022 Tuesday

Here I realized I was keeping this log for more than just my daily references...

Went back to two Valacyclovir today. as per doctor request (I had been taking three per day, 1500mg total, but research literature had recommended long term for 2,000mg per day for some clients like myself).

Went to Winco (local employee owned supermarket with the cheapest prices around, but still quality foods).

Evening, had sinus headache of the type I get when I contracted COVID.

Worked to open sinuses using all day saline flushing (half hour and/or hourly), took antihistamines.

18 May 2022 Wednesday

In morning, felt better, no sinus headache.

Woke feeling foggy again and took a pill.

VA hosp called for ultrasound, I called them back immediately after at noon and supplied my info on voicemail, requesting American Lake Puget Sound VA Hospital location (not Seattle, which requires a ferry ride from Bremerton, and dealing with Seattle traffic). I waited for callback.

2:30PM I got scheduled for Thursday July 14th, 11am. Fast for 6-8 hours, I can drink plain coffee/tea, take water/meds/vits. Go to Building 81, 2nd floor.

3PM Took another pill

11PM Another pill

Felt weird all day. Am I fighting off ANOTHER new covid infection?

Finally got a twenty min walk in, in the sun, and it felt great!

Again felt weird all afternoon, maybe due to not taking three Valacyclovir per day?

19 May 2022 Thursday

Woke after a night of sleep difficulty, didn't get enough sleep, but don't feel too bad.

Woke feeling I needed to continue so three pills today.

Lungs are "wet", as if I did catch something, and it dropped into my lungs. Been there, done that, got that damn T-shirt!

Took covid home test (ordered eight free from government yesterday via USPS).

Covid test was negative, but sure feels like I caught it again. Light symptoms, but lung issues are always scary for what they can portend.

Took Valacyclovir in morning 8AM and I think it helped. Also took half a chlorpheniramine maleate (old generation 1 antihistamine that I've been taking most of my life and first found in the cold med "Contact". Just after high school in my first job (with poor ventilation in the sub-sub basement) I found Contact helped me, but also knocked me out. So I took apart the capsules wondering at the different colored spheres. I looked up the med ingredients listed on the pack and spent the next few months zeroing in on which drug/chemical helped me. It turned out to be a yellow pill... chlorpheniramine maleate. All my life, either (and/or) that and Sudafed have been most helpful to me, I could get through the allergy season. In trying nasal sprays, I'd need them so much I found I would get what I eventually discovered was "rebound" effect, where you'd get relief from the spray, then it would make you sick again anyway and in another way. You could also get addicted to it. (see ref# 26)

20 May 2022 Friday

Slept, waking up repeatedly, BUT was able to go right back to sleep. So woke fairly rested.

After I got up, felt ill overall, sinuses congested.

Flushing & used nasal spray (used Simvillasan natural sinus spray that my Yoga instructor cousin turned me onto), which helped with sinuses.

Benadryl helped with the overall ill LC feeling.

4PM Felt better

21 May 2022 Saturday

6AM Woke. Could have used more sleep but slept OK, mostly.

Woke feeling good and wasn't going to take a pill.

Felt almost like covid is over for me. By breakfast I could still feel it was there, however.

But maybe I'm nearing the end? (uh huh, sure, sure ya are...)

I feel I could stop taking Valacyclovir now, but I will take it at 8AM and maybe that will be the last, taking one more than one needs, to end with?

10AM I started feeling bad again, slightly, but obvious what it was and that it was coming back, so I took another Valacyclovir.

Took a Valacyclovir at bedtime.

22 May 2022 Sunday

8AM Got up. Felt tired, kind of crummy when I woke up, but slept through the night for a change. No Valacyclovir in the morning. If the illness increases over the day I'll take more, but I may be able to stop now. Hoping I start feeling better from here on. But I will have to wait till about 11AM (I went to bed around that time last night...11PM), in order to see whats what after the pill wears off.

23 May 2022 Monday

Added 1000mg Vit C a day extra, as I read the virus doesn't like it [this is where I found that article about Vit. C therapy for Herpes virus]

Feeling good off the Valacyclovir. Still feeling the virus, but getting better. Going for walks, longer each day.

9:30AM Feeling my heartbeat (I prefer not to, as it can mean pulse or BP are rising or have risen) and wondered if in being off Valacyclovir, it gives the virus time to build back up? Or if I'm still fighting it off to its end, (hopefully) soon. Feeling still the overall body feel of a virus lingering.

24 May 2022 Tuesday

Woke and feel the virus & higher BP than normal. I feel I should be taking Valacyclovir...am I allowing the viral load to increase by not taking it? Will this ever go away? Please?

I feel like not taking the pills is allowing viral load to increase and I can now feel it affecting my blood pressure...again. Damn!

7:45AM BP: 130 / 70

7:46AM 122/76 p80 BP got better eventually.

11:20AM Taking Vit C 1000mg 5x daily to see if it helps as it can apparently help with some herpes virus issues, at 8am, 11:30AM, 2:30PM, 5:30PM, 8:30PM.

25 May 2022 Wednesday

Slept OK, Woke once or twice mid-night feeling heart/BP issues.

Calmed myself and fell asleep. It feels like in not being on the Valacyclovir it allows for these heart issues. I can't help wondering if I'm doing my body damage in allowing the virus, or for it to increase and sustain over time? I know what the doctor says, but if he's wrong, I die? Or become damaged? It's not his fault, but our overall lack of info still, on this. How many have we already lost to our ignorance on this? 1,000s and 1,000s? 100,000s?

Woke feeling tired and this damned virus (hate this overall body ill feeling), bit of sinus pain.

Took 1000 mg vit. c. 8AM, 12noon, 3PM, 6PM, 9PM

The Vit C mega-dosing seems to help tamp down symptoms, which are mostly an overall body feeling of discomfort. Had a Blood Pressure incident that lasted twenty minutes or so in early evening.

1:37PM BP 121/69 p87

Each day I'm using between half a Benadryl and/or half a chlorpheniramine maleate that seem to help.

Went to go for a walk but BP felt above normal. Took half a chlorpheniramine maleate and felt better. Is the Benadryl not working, or do I just need to take a whole one? [I discovered that frequently I wasn't taking enough Benadryl]

No walk today.

26 May 2022 Thursday

Woke feeling a bit tired, but the best I've felt in a while. As perhaps the virus is fading (from the Vit C?)?

Took 1000mg Vit. C, at 7:30AM, 11:30AM, 3:30PM, 6PM, 7PM, 10PM (2000mg for entire night).

9:48AM Feeling a bit weird today. Maybe breakfast, toaster

waffles & sausage and espresso. BP spiked, took a chlorpheniramine maleate (half pill as usual) and did calming breathing exercises and felt better

Tomorrow something more substantial/reasonable. Also, woke a bit congested, seasonal allergies lately have been a problem with this weather changing so much. I swear, PNW weather is going to be the death of me. :)

9:55AM took another half CM pill, ate some nuts.

Allergies are bad today/this week. Took half a Benadryl about 11AM.

27 May 2022 Friday

Woke in the night with tachycardia, calmed and fell back asleep, manageable but disturbing.

No Vit C mega dosing today, just an extra 500mg single Vit with normal morning Vits today

Feeling overall uncomfortable.

Emailed VA Doc about links, research and my situation.

Took half a Benadryl about 11AM and felt overall way better, oddly enough. As if it's a histamine reaction I'm feeling...in part anyway. [this turns out later to be significant after the doctor said it's more likely the calming effect of Benadryl, which wasn't the case, or if so, not significantly.]

29 May 2022 Saturday

Slept OK. Woke with sharp upper sinus pain which has been coming on for a couple of days. It only takes a day or two of sinuses being closed for infection to begin, that according to my pre VA Doctor years ago who turned me onto saline flushing. Sometimes I've had to use a lot of decongestants and antihistamines and saline flushing to open and clear an infection, usually flushing hourly, for three days.

Day 1 of 2nd set of mega dosing Vit C for three days. If I knocked down the virus this much, maybe again will deactivate it? Sinus flush hourly all day. Overall crummy body feeling from virus, or something.

29 May 2022 Sunday

Slept through the night, woke feeling the best I have in a while!

Day 2 of 2nd set of doing Vit C mega dosing. 7:30AM, 10:30AM, 2PM, 5:30PM, 9:30PM.

Continuing Benadryl & Chlor. Maleate (half pills each, at a time) and hourly sinus flushing.

7:30AM Had one toaster waffle & maple syrup and two Jimmy Dean sausage patties and a double shot of espresso (normal is two doubles but it's been untenable these two months of illness as it raises my BP or pulse uncomfortably). Shortly after, 15-20mins, blood pressure went up a bit. Relaxed, breathed, and got BP down.

About 8:30AM starting noticing overall body ill, as if the virus was again noticeable.

Antihistamines do seem to help a bit.

2:10PM Blood pressure spiked pretty good. Took fifteen minutes to breathe it back to fairly normal, and was a bit spooky. Took half a Benadryl. Can't help but wonder if it's because I'm not taking anti virals, allowing the virus to be there at any level and, what damage may it be causing, long term? That's the scary thing in all this, the unknowables, years down the road (or worse, months?).

4:45PM Started to feel the "virus" or whatever, overwhelming my body. It got disturbing. I took half a Chlor. Maleate and felt better from it.

6:30PM Felt overwhelmed with the virus, like it's growing and affecting my BP/heart rate, etc. Then after about fifteen minutes, it passed. As if these last two instances of growth were a "bloom" as it fights the Vit C and then...as happened last week with this regimen, it lost. The "attacking dying animal syndrome" as it fights any or all, as it dies. I've noticed this with illness before. Just before the "fever breaks" it gets really bad, then just vanishes.

Feeling better now, lighter. It was a little scary (what if Vit C grew the virus and it was about to kill me? But I KNEW that's not it as I'd done this last week. It worked then, as it did tonight).

As happens with some illnesses, it gets really bad before it then just, dies off.

7:43PM Another flare up like above two. Hate these. This was less? About a minute.

30 May 2022 Monday Memorial Day

Last day Vit C mega dosing for three day schedule. Fell asleep around 11:30PM or so.

Woke a little tired, about 5AM, about thirty minutes of seemingly arrhythmic tachycardia and slightly higher BP.

Vit C: 7:30AM, 11AM, 3PM, 7PM, 11PM.

31 May 2022 Tuesday

Slept through the night. Woke with my heart beating OK but kind of odd feeling.

I can feel the virus all the time, all over and I hate that. I want to feel normal again.

Dropped down to Vit C 1000mg per meal, maybe one at bedtime.

Went for a short walk outside about 11AM. Wasn't feeling 100%, but got in some steps. Maybe half of usual, much less than last time.

2PM Feeling pretty good about now.

Bad trouble getting to sleep. Bowel & urinary discomfort after having go to the bathroom before I could fall asleep (had to get up when I realized that).

Feeling scalp pain (BP headache) off and on today, and totally relaxing helped it go away & lower BP.

Again wondering if the Vit C use is helping, but still allowing viral issues to affect or damage my system. Rather than using anti virals as I would like to be doing. Noticed when I was consciously "relaxing" my body to fall asleep, I wasn't actually as relaxed as I'd thought. There was tension in my muscles in places I didn't expect to notice it. Forcing relaxation calmed my pulse/BP and eventually I fell asleep and slept until I woke in the morning.

Wondering if this form of Vit C at this dose is causing digestive problems and another form of Vit C might be better?

1 June 2022 Wednesday

Woke feeling somewhat exhausted, not feeling great, feeling BP issues, scalp discomfort/almost pain. Why am I so easily tensing up my body to raise BP? I think the Vit C is tearing up my insides [it can normally in high doses, do that]. After a half a Benadryl, I felt better (though still tired), by just before 10AM.

12:30AM Trouble going to sleep, still awake

2 June 2022 Thursday

5:30AM Woke with high blood pressure, heart throbbing, headache. Tried breathing exercises in bed, to no effect. Got up, drank water, took half a Benadryl, back to bed (to try to sleep more). Did breathing exercises until BP went down. Couldn't sleep (for yet another morning...) so got up but... felt the best I have in a while. Still feel the virus, but is the Vit C thing working now?

3 June 2022 Friday

(eldest son's birthday)

Had trouble getting to sleep again. Woke too early with blood pressure high. Did breathing which helped a little. Got up & drank cold water and took half a Benadryl. Back to bed and breathing exercises. Fell asleep for an hour or so and woke feeling BP more normal. Feel pretty tired (not as bad as yesterday) and just crummy. Heart beating oddly, feels like BP is now too low or something. But probably just from being tired. Eyes started being rough, like sand in them for some reason.

Emailed VA Doctor to ask again for the Valacyclovir. It's frustrating finding doctors publishing good results they have with patients going through what you are, but you can't convince anyone else. Especially, when you try it and it works!

4 June 2022 Saturday

After feeling worse all week, today I woke feeling horrible. Like energy was draining and I was hollow or something. Horrible feeling. In a way, it felt like I was slowly dying. This disease has a never ending variety of how to make one feel bad. It feels like it's dropping into my stomach/intestines which is scary. As that can lead to some very bad issues according to the medical literature. Found research that certain types of stomach problems from LC can lead to death... in months. But most people don't/won't get that. So, probably not me!

By 9AM I'd had it. I took a Valacyclovir. Within THREE hours I noticed I felt a little better. I did not feel well all day but by afternoon it felt like I might be feeling better. By evening I knew I was feeling better. I took a second pill at 9PM. Eyes were even more like they had sand in them. Never had that before and I really don't like it. What is that? So much the uncomfortableness of these many new feelings/issues from LC are because you don't know what they mean. Or if it's something far worse than you might believe.

5 June 2022 Sunday

Woke after a couple of hours, fell asleep, woke four hour later. Felt more rested today. Bit of a sinus headache, took half a Chlor. Maleate, drank some water and went back to bed. Dozed a bit and got up. The overall ill feeling is gone that I was experiencing this past week, but I'm feeling my heart beating in uncomfortable ways. Hoping taking the next Valacyclovir will help, and eating breakfast, as food does tend to help me feel better whenever it's past time to eat.

8PM For a time as I write this, I feel perfectly normal. Not so an hour ago. That lasted about ten minutes. But, it's progress. Eyes were bad like sand in them. Nothing helps, but used allergy drops a few times today and kept them well moistened, as I always do but now even more so. I do have a condition where the surface of my eyes wrinkles a bit (conjunctivochalasis, maybe, a condition that causes the conjunctiva, the clear tissue layer that covers the eye, to loosen, wrinkle, and fold), making vision problematic, mostly at night and when driving it can be dangerous. Eye doctor has me taking a 5% saline solution eye drop, three times a day (forever, apparently). It helps a lot to make the eye surface lay down. As does never letting my eyes dry out and keeping artificial tears always at hand. Mostly, it's not much of an issue.

6 June 2022 Monday

Slept most the night, woke feeling pretty good. A bit of the virus feel until I was up for a bit. Better after breakfast (oatmeal). Eyes feel fine today. That was so odd, feeling like sand in the eyes.

As I showered at 9AM today, I realized I felt normal for the first time since stopping Valacyclovir a while back. VA Doctor today refused me any more Valacyclovir. After shower I sat down, rested and BP was up a bit, but then went back down.

I've noticed at the worst times in this condition, that after showering my pulse/BP is up too high. Is that the physical action of showering, or the hot water, which feels so good? I know cold water helps this issue decrease, as with drinking cold water, or lesser so splashing it one's face.

Felt not so great before lunch, but pretty good after eating & taking Vit C.

Not feeling the overall crumminess, but feeling odd, like feeling the virus throughout my nervous system. Maybe what it feels like to have MS, almost, like I'm going to start shaking all over, but don't.

I have an idea...

I'll take a Valacyclovir pill tonight, but then, just a pill every night to stretch it and maybe guarantee me a good night's sleep? If only... [this is not so much how this medicine works]

Below is the response from the VA infectious disease physician:

"Thank you for the interesting consult and observation. We are unaware of any guidelines or trials that suggest a role of Valacyclovir in the treatment of Long Covid syndrome. Currently based on CDC and NIH guidelines and guidance

Valacyclovir has not been listed as a medication for the treatment of COVID19. We sincerely don't have an explanation for the relationship between use of Valacyclovir and symptom relief of long covid syndrome."
No mention was made they would like to evaluate me in person or through telemedicine, so no additional referral had been made at that time.

My Response:

"Thank you, for the quick update. Curious.
"As I'm obviously suffering through something that presents as long covid, it would be nice to find some medical relief to the condition.
"Alas... I can only hope as happened previously, that it will eventually burn itself out. Hopefully before it burns me out, as I prefer to outlast it. Though I do realize, some do not.
"The CDC is still collecting and revising data, but NCHS has so far identified 60 death certificates that list long covid or similar terminology — for example, "post-covid" — in 2021 and another 60 during the first five months of 2022."
"Since I've had it before and it went away, though this version is far more intrusive and abusive, I will simply hope to eventually outlast it.
"Have a nice week."

7 June 2022 Tuesday

Slept through the night until 5:30AM, but woke with elevated blood pressure and a slight sinus headache. Got up, drank water, hesitantly took half a Benadryl. Within fifteen minutes I could feel my body & sinuses opening up, hypertension went down, didn't feel my heart beating anymore and felt much better. Is my body allergic to itself, or what? Histamines causing higher blood pressure? Is my immune system attacking my nervous system?

After I got up, I felt... not so great. No Valacyclovir until bedtime. Wondering if I should skip it (did the combo of that and mega dosing Vit C help things?).

75 degrees out today. Was able to do some chores outside, slowly cleaned the driveway, mowed the small parking strip. Maybe mow the yard tomorrow when it's to be cooler? Heat makes any exercise as if I were doing much more than I am.

8 June 2022 Wednesday

Got 2nd booster shot at Safeway because at yesterday's VA teleconference town hall meeting, they indicated my cohort/age should get one. So I now have had two Pfizer shots, one Pfizer booster and one Moderna booster. And I have stock in Pfizer and Lily, which I thought would work out well these past two years. But it was the stock in Ely Lily stock that actually did incredible. [later I heard about a lawsuit by Moderna on Phizer and sold that stock before it decreased any in value]

9 June 2022 Thursday

Felt pretty good after booster yesterday. It's odd sleeping through the night now.

10 June 2022 Friday

Woke only once with BP issues, breathing technique to lower it enough to get back to sleep.

Woke feeling a little uncomfortable with increased issues that had been on the decline. I believe evoked by the booster shot. Some pulse & BP issues. [that also happened at my next updated booster on a Monday where I was not well all week and then Saturday morning felt much better]

Felt good enough to do wash, not just one load, but two. Which has been unusual. Washed both clothes and sheets.

11 June 2022 Saturday

Slept through the night, woke feeling tired and that higher "viral load" feeling. Thought of taking Valacyclovir but did not. Same as yesterday, woke feeling uncomfortable but better than yesterday with booster invoked issues decreasing.

It feels like I may be getting over the LC. [uh...no.]

Walked to 19th St. (0.6 mile) and back (1.2 miles).

12 June 2022 Sunday

Sick of feeling sick. Took a Valacyclovir at bedtime.

13 June 2022 Monday

Fitful sleep, tired in the morning. Took two Valacyclovir today. Wondered if I was screwing up as I feel worse today [that might be from the exercise]. But made it to drive to Safeway for groceries. Sinus congestion today, taking Benadryl (it's helped so much getting me through this disease, esp. lately when I want to take a Valacyclovir but don't, when my heart starts beating weird, or BP goes up). If I take half a Benadryl, it returns to normal in fifteen minutes or so.

14 June 2022 Tuesday

Oh my god! Woke feeling almost normal!

I can feel the virus at a very low level, just humming along. What a god send, and I'm not even religious! Have high hopes.

VA doctor thinks what, I'm insane? Lying? Stupid? Perhaps he's right and Valacyclovir does not work on covid (I know that's true) or on long covid (I have to wonder about that, as it sure seems to work). Perhaps this is not long covid but just activated herpes virus, or a virus Valacyclovir DOES work on because... It is OBVIOUSLY working for some reason!

Took two Valacyclovir today, last one is tomorrow morning.

15 June 2022 Wednesday

Last Valacyclovir in morning for this normal schedule of two pills a day, three day cycle of meds.

16 June 2022 Thursday

Slept through the night, woke only once, for a moment. A bit frightened that I felt normal for once and it would probably, or might, return to the long covid feelings.

By 7:30AM I could again feel the long covid a bit in the background, but hoping it fades.

Felt worse over the next few hours, but not what I would say horrible, as previous, even last week.

If I had to guess, I'd say maybe another three months of this long covid. Or it could just go away tomorrow. Maybe six months? It seems to use the half life method of dissolution in never seeming to go away until it finally is gone, as it takes (seemingly) forever.

17 June 2022 Friday

Woke feeling the long covid again.

9:30AM Had productive teleMed meeting with VA doctor who said he'd have a specialist look at my records about long covid and OK'd a thirty day course of Valacyclovir (1000mg in morning, or 2/500mg 2x a day). Success! Relief!

Took two of my extra Valacyclovir laying around (as I had them, but told the doctor I'd stop as he wished) to jump start it, at about 10AM. Felt BP up (told Doc it was 124/74 pulse 82 just before telemed appt). Half a Benadryl to help lower BP.

This weather is giving me sinus allergy grief. Is the LC exacerbating that? Seems like it.

18 June 2022 Saturday

First day post doc appt of authorized twice daily use of 500mg of Valacyclovir.

Woke feeling virusy but better than yesterday. Nervous system wasn't "humming" as it was yesterday so uncomfortably, but an overall "yuck" feeling.

Wanted to take a Valacyclovir upon rising but tried to push it until the normal 9AM time. Took a chlor. maleate (half of 2mg pill) and it helped.

9AM Took Valacyclovir pill. Felt pretty crummy after that for a while. Started feeling better around noon, maybe sooner.

3:30PM Feel not too bad now. When I move around more I feel it's still there, but sitting still it's OK. Looking forward to another day or so of the pills under my belt to where the viral load or whatever is lower and more manageable.

9PM Took next pill

11PM feeling pretty good

19 June 2022 Sunday - Father's Day

Trouble getting to sleep, kept waking up.

4AM woke wide, with seemingly irregular heart beat for a while. Finally fell asleep after a while, for a bit. Woke several times.

7:30AM Finally up feeling somewhat exhausted. BP still a bit higher than I'd like. So sick of this stupid condition after almost three months now.

20 June 2022 Monday

Fitful sleep again, heart beating weirdly again. Woke tired but felt way less viral load today.

Three days of daily Valacyclovir and I'm feeling the positive effects FINALLY...I think.

The past three days have been very uncomfortable, but that happens when restarting the Valacyclovir.

Thought I'd try mowing some of my now almost 4' high lawn, finally feeling well enough to consider it. Got the mower out but the battery was dead. So I started it charging and gave up for today.

Overall feeling kind of weird today, maybe BP? Thought maybe it was unusually low? So I took it:

12:28PM BP 124/69 95 pulse. Nope, not low. Nuts. I think...

12:33PM Would too low be better than too high? Sigh... BP 120/65 91 pulse

It seems whenever I start to feel better in one way, this thing comes up with a new way to define uncomfortable.

3:30PM That really crummy feeling I was experiencing seemed to pass, mostly.

1:30AM Trouble getting to sleep, finally slept through the night.

21 June 2022 Tuesday First day of Summer

7AM Woke with slight sinus headache and BP higher than I'd like. Did a few minutes breathing exercises, then massaged vagus nerve around ear (which seemed to do the trick). Sinuses tension/pain relaxed at that point too, which was interesting.

https://drruscio.com/vagus-nerve-massage/

9AM Emailed VA doctor to be sure script was submitted.

I'm really sick of this very disturbing disease! Not to mention our lack of medical help for it.

At almost noon I felt a slight pain down to the tips of my fingers of my left hand. It's hard to define this as a heart issue and this has happened many times these past three months since contracting this. I've had sustained numbness of my left hand's fingers and tingling like needles going on too long. For this occurrence it could just be from exercising, using my left arm too much (why no pain on the right?) on lawn mowing a 3-4' tall lawn.

So I broke down and trying not to do much today. Took half a Benadryl. I also can't tell if that made the pain go away or just moving it around did it. It wasn't profound enough to be of real concern or call anyone about it. I ate lunch just after noon time and that usually makes me feel better over all, getting some protein into me (I'd had oatmeal as usual for breakfast, and in mid morning, some nuts).

My email response today to my VA doctor after being refused long term Valicyclovir treatment

(I was later allowed a one time 30 day supply. When that ran out I requested another 30 day supply anyway, including information/data indicating it was effective and it was eventually supplied. I asked for no more after that. [I finally got the 30 day supply and then oddly, another a week later]

"Hi, I just wanted to note a couple of things. No need for a response.
I worry if I don't use the Valicyclovir, which is keeping symptoms down of I assume the herpes virus in some form, what damage to my metabolism may it be doing during that time?
Once the Valacyclovir is working for me, my blood pressure being intermittently a bit high, seems to be my primary concern that bothers me.
The other thing is... how many people, as statistically I cannot be the only one, are going through what I am and don't know this med helps, and they could be helped by it.
Or those who do realize it, that the Valacyclovir helps, but give up when told it doesn't or won't work, or simply hit a wall in trying to get it and are of such a depleted state of mind, they just give up and continue to suffer with it?
I think those are valid concerns, but not just for me, but how many others?
Thanks, that's it."
The information/data I supplied later to request a second 30 day supply (included here elsewhere), stated that I went on Valacyclovir for several weeks, came off it and was good for

THREE WEEKS without it and feeling good. Then going back on it for three days, a normal schedule for a herpes outbreak, and then stayed off of it for two weeks, before needing it again, and before the long covid viral load increased enough to be very uncomfortable. I then did another three days on it which lasted without it for one week. Three weeks off, two weeks off, one week off. Indicating to me that long term use was indicated and preferable.

And so I was supplied another 30 day supply.

12:42PM

Pain end of finger tips returned. Little finger & ring finger. Wondering if it's a pinched nerve in my armpit or something. Received the VA disease specialist's comments (shared here elsewhere), and VA Doctor shared it with me. Basically useless comments, other than that I'm an interesting case and no one knows about Valacyclovir being effective. Although, as I'd pointed out, they do. Sigh.

I responded, again saying I can't be the only one like this and what damage may be, being done to my body in my not being on the med?

22 June 2022 Wednesday

Miserable night due to blood pressure. Woke several times because of it until I was lying there for ten minutes, about 2:30AM, breathing, trying to lower it. Gave up, took half a Benadryl. Which didn't seem to help.

3:30AM Woke still with BP issue. Fell asleep.

4:20AM Woke feeling better. Fell asleep.

7AM Woke and got up feeling exhausted. Could this be from mowing the lawn? As I do tend toward allergy issues after mowing, though I wore a mask which helped. Also, exercise can cause issues.

The exercise/mowing yesterday felt great. Though I had to stop three times to let my BP go back to normal. So, were the BP issues all last evening due to allergies to the mowing, or the exercise?

I've read in the medical lit that covid or long covid can be helped to decrease with exercise. Or at times... it enhances the disease, depending on what is going on. Not, helpful. So exercise helps you or hurts you with LC. Great. I'm seeing so much information like that in the medical literature, too.

2PM I feel like this might be the baseline for the best I'll feel on Valacyclovir until I get over this long covid crap.

Slight headache. Front/temples today, that comes and goes, carrying over from yesterday afternoon.

23 June 2022 Thursday

Slept OK, waking once feeling BP. Fell asleep quickly, woke feeling tired, nonetheless.

So sick of getting older, as well as this damn illness!

WALKED more briskly than since I got sick, from home to 19th St (.6 mile) and back to my street (.5 mile, then back to 19th (.5 mile) and home (.6 mile), about 2.2 miles. The most I've walked this year & since contracting this on March 28th.

I'm tired but it felt great the entire time, as well as now. My thoughts now are to get as much exercise as I can to shorten this illness, according to that potential from my readings on long covid, etc. Some say exercise can be bad, but my gut says that more may do more good than harm. But overdoing it could be bad.

24 June 2022 Friday

2AM Woke to relieve myself... a lot.

5:30AM Woke with heart beating, high BP, breathing to calm it. Could feel the covid strongly humming all over my body. Felt despair over it...how can I go on with this ANY longer? I'm sick of being sick!

Laid there not dozing, but almost, with NPR on.

7AM Put on Elton John's "Madman Across the Water" (seemed appropriate) and started to feel better. 7:15AM Got up feeling better. covid backed off, despair already gone. As if during sleep the covid wakes up more, as the literature I read yesterday indicates, and that the immune system is stronger during the day. Also, cortisol levels are lower at night (Cortisol production drops to its lowest point around midnight).

Found the Facebook Long Covid support group
https://www.facebook.com/LongCovidPage

People there talk a lot about histamines and treatment oriented around a low histamine diet, etc.

Oh? Which would explain why when I ate something/somethings, after I'd eat I'd have BP issues. And when I take Benadryl it helps reduce BP. VA doctor had conjectured that it may just be the calming effect one can get from Benadryl as a side effect. Uh, maybe not so much. I never bought that as what was going on, but told him on the phone once...

"Sure, but it's for reducing the effects of histamines and that just seems more like what is going on."
Basically not just histamine levels, but it also involves raising your blood sugar levels when some foods increase that, which histamines can also do. So stopping the honey I've been using, etc.

Found "Healing Histamine", started learning about high/low level histamine foods:

https://healinghistamine.com/what-is-histamine/

25 June 2022 Saturday

Trouble getting to sleep, slept through the night, got up to relieve myself (a lot).

4:30AM Woke and dozed until...

6AM, turned on NPR.

Before, my BP would intermittently spike after eating. Now as I pay attention to eating low histamine foods, it's no longer spiking after eating, which is rather nice.

Took half a melatonin at bed time to test if it raised my BP. I had found a reference saying it can, at times. But as the VA doctor said, when that happened, it was probably just a coincidence. And that time I believe, he might be right.

26 June 2022 Sunday

Seems doctor was right. Melatonin worked great. Slept through the night, woke too early. I could feel the virus and it took a long time to want to get out of bed.

Walked 2.2 miles today, early before it got too hot.

Stopped by home to take my now late 9AM Valacyclovir and was going to go do another mile but didn't. Maybe next time, if it wasn't already too hot at only 74 degrees out.

Supposed to get up to 90 today.

10:17AM 82 degrees.

5:15pm BP 124/73BPM 86 pulse

It seems the more I exercise the less I need Benadryl to lower BP.

Ate dinner with high sodium 900mg, chicken Kiev/bacon wrapped, to see if I get a BP reaction. As high sodium seems to raise my BP a lot.

27 June 2022 Monday

Couldn't get to sleep, had trouble sleeping.

3AM Woke with high BP, took half Benadryl.

4:30AM Woke, took half Benadryl.

7AM Got up, took half Benadryl. Had breakfast, 2 fried eggs & toast. Took half Benadryl and half chlor. maleate and BP calmed down.

Too tired to hit Costco today in Silverdale, 11 miles away.

Looked it up, bacon has lots of histamine, as did the chicken Kiev last night. Which even tasted too salty, not bad, but I didn't need that much sodium. So it did cause me a bigger need for antihistamine.

Wish I hadn't eaten it. Figured after hitting the bathroom, I'd feel better, though O felt better before that, I think I did feel better after, too. Once the chicken Kiev was fully out of my system.

Valacylovir 30 day script from VA should arrive today.

Feeling pretty crummy all day, apparently from triggering long covid with high histamine/sodium levels for dinner yesterday. I seem to tolerate 5-600mg sodium well, but between that and 900mg, there seems to be a cut off point. But is it per day, or per meal?

Ate a bag of microwave popcorn, was this bad to do, too? I did this last week with no affect from the salt, etc.

28 June 2022 Tuesday

11:30PM Uncomfortable BP issues. Little bit hard getting to sleep. Tried breathing exercise for a while. Finally got up, relieved myself, took an entire Benadryl. Once I fell asleep, mostly slept through the night, waking up feeling different.

6AM Got up, tired, but not exhausted. Feeling...better? Wondering if this was my actions in eating high histamine/salt, or am I nearing the death of this thing (LC)? [again, nope, dream on]

I wonder if the past two days were yet another long covid flare up (as I've seen before these past three months to be sure) indicating my meds, Vit C & exercise (and maybe diet?) are working and this isn't a shift to another (lower?) level now.

I did it! 3.5 mile walk today (6 lengths up and back to 19th St)!

29 June 2022 Wednesday

Horrible night again. Couldn't get to sleep.

12:30AM broke down and took half a melatonin. Woke too early with too little sleep, not feeling well. Maybe I have a sinus infection on top of long covid now. Oh joy. Lied there in bed listening to NPR for a couple of hours, in and out sleep. Weird dreams.

Start flushing sinuses a lot today. Planned to go to Costco today but ...nope.

Interesting thought, as when you start to exercise, esp. to lose weight, it can make you ill. But you just have to keep going where so many will just stop. As with this, maybe in my doing 3.5 miles walking yesterday... what, I get a bad night of sleep and wake up feeling sick? Nice.

On the other hand, seasonal allergy changes have been rampant with weather changes which also affect me annually so...shut up, stop complaining and just keep exercising!

Wasn't getting to sleep quickly at 10:10PM after I got to bed.

Midnight. I took half a melatonin. Then slept well.

30 June 2022 Thursday

Woke feeling tired, but not exhausted. More rested than all week. After I finally got up after listening to NPR for a long time, feeling the virus, I felt better than worse.

I know, weird observations.

Was going to Silverdale to the art/frame store & Costco today, but decided to wait until after the holiday weekend.

Wasn't getting to sleep, tired as I was, so took half a melatonin.

1 July 2022 Friday

Woke feeling pretty good. French toast for breakfast. Was going to shoot for walking five miles today though I knew I should skip a day, due to my left ankle pain. Got in three laps, 3.2 miles. Foot was hurting bad enough to stop there. Iced it, put cannabis salve on it.

Overall, feeling better today, virus wise.

2 July 2022 Saturday

Started shooting for 10PM bedtimes due to article about healing via circadian rhythm.

Took a melatonin to sleep, couldn't get to sleep. Had interesting dreams, woke feeling, not too bad. Ankle felt good today

Made it walking five miles today, five laps up to 19th St. and back. Yay! Ankle hurt at the beginning of lap five, but after half a block or so it didn't hurt any more. 2.5 hours of walking, 11,284 steps today.

1:30PM Ate an air fried half chicken for a late lunch along with some hummus & broccoli. Hummus histamine wise is supposed to be problematic, but seems OK.

Looked up lentils for histamines and found they are problematic. But the cans of lentil soup from Costco seemed OK, so far. Tried the veggie lentil soup version for dinner. Ate a little and waited for reaction before trying more. So far so good.

After dinner I ate a shortbread cookie (sugar) and a square of chocolate (sugar) and my BP didn't go up as before. Only a tiny bit, indicating perhaps, healing? Maybe. My efforts in exercise are working?

10:17PM. Got into bed. Could not get to sleep. Took partial, then entire melatonin pill. To no effect.

1:30AM took a Benadryl, I could still feel my heart pounding a little in my chest.

3 July 2022 Sunday

Woke tired, feeling my vagus nerve (perhaps) irritated, though healing now, maybe from something aggravating it? Vagus nerve feeling is a feeling from neck (higher when it's bad) down through body center to belly button area. It's, odd.

I have to assume this was either walking the five miles for the first time in a while yesterday, or the sugar/lentils I ate after they hit my small intestines, or passed my duodenum. Or both. I have to try this again, lentils anyway. And after no exercise that day, just to see if that was the issue.

11AM Not feeling as healed as yesterday, sadly. Assuming it was, if not the over exercise, pushing that, which is needed, maybe it was the sugar & lentils?

According to my readings:

"Histamine is a natural product of the decomposition of the amino acid Histidine. Amino acids are the building blocks of proteins: So wherever proteins are present, there also is histamine."

https://food.r-biopharm.com/news/histamine-intolerance-fish/

Received Organic India Tulsi tea today and started drinking a tea bag worth a day ("For maximum health benefits, drink three to five cups daily...though even one cup of Tulsi Tea a day is beneficial."). Maybe slightly beneficial but at this point, anything is helpful/welcome.

Sugar seems to be an issue for me. So maybe for now, alcohol too, and histamines. Except some high histamine foods (eggs, shrimp, others) don't seem to bother me. So it must be something about or around histamines.

Took a full melatonin at bedtime.

4th of July 2022 Monday

Slept through the night, woke too early, dozed.

7AM Got up.

Feeling the virus again today. Either because of the five miles the other day, or eating too much histamine & sugar that day. Sucks, man...

Later.. not having a good long covid day. Maybe I got too cocky on Saturday with the five miles and eating almost normally...

5 July 2022 Tuesday

Felt the vagus nerve too much.

Hit Costco after frame shop in Silverdale, about my new wood block print. I didn't feel great, but got through Costco.

6 July 2022 Wednesday

6:30AM Slept OK. Got up.

Feeling the virus too much, but it's doable. Feeling better today regarding the vagus nerve. Perhaps healing from the five mile over do last Saturday. I know the warning signs now, while walking. Next time I'll quit before going too far. Last time, the last half mile my entire left arm was aching. Which was just, odd. Creepy.

7 July 2022 Thursday

Slept well (again without melatonin). Woke with sinus pain, the virus feeling there, but lighter. Am I getting over it, finally. [spoiler...Nope] Or is this more "half life demise syndrome", where I'll feel it there as it lessens months after month [pretty much]? My first feeling was did I catch another "flavor" of covid in going to Costco, Tuesday? Or is this another viral death throe where finally I'm seeing progress [could be]?

3PM A visual migraine was starting up. But the visuals, which for decades (the few times I have had migraines) have begun with blindness building in the center of my visual range. Then a halo of colors appear. But now it's an overall kind of affect to my visual range. The colors begin in my lower range, just left of center visual field and projects upward in a curve, going toward the center top. Strange.

Took half a chlorpheniramine maleate, which usually does the trick (unless it's bad, then a whole tablet, unless it's really bad, then pretty much nothing works). Then half a Benadryl, as it felt a little too intense. Then took the other half of CM tab.

I'M SURE THIS IS NONSENSE but...I am wondering if I'm getting over long covid today. It kind of feels like it. I'm eating cookies with sugar in them as tests and my body isn't freaking out (yet). Testing the virus diminishing, I ate too freely (sugar mostly) and too late. So at bedtime I worried a bit.

Took a melatonin at bedtime just to be sure.

8 July 2022 Friday

Woke feeling a little tired. Probably due to slight BP issues. Had very weird dreams, esp. one about being in Hawaii with my late mother, family and friends. I was bitten in a hotel room when changing, by a spider (or tiny bird?). I couldn't extract it before it bit me, even though I was bitten (hey, it's a dream, it has to make sense?).

The middle of my hand swelled up in a blister and... I woke. Maybe because yesterday afternoon I accidentally bit my inner left cheek resulting in a blood blister. Never had that happen in my mouth before. I popped it with a sterilized pin and spit blood. Gross. It was a bit sore, even the next morning. Maybe somehow that affected my dream? But in the dream it was on my hand.

Woke again with sinus headache, but still lighter viral feel than days ago. Did not wake with bad BP issues, but had a slight bit of heartbeat being too "loud" in my chest. So I got up and took half a melatonin and got back to sleep. Later woke without that feeling.

Wondering if the Tulsi tea is helping. I'd been drinking it for three days when I started feeling better after the Saturday five mile debacle. Though I'm only doing a tea bag a day, not 3-5 as recommended.

9 July 2022 Saturday

Woke a bit tired, but slept through the night without a melatonin.

I can feel the virus, as it's still there, more than I felt it yesterday. So my hopes of it almost being gone, are dashed a bit.

Didn't feel that great to walk today, though I should.

I did end up doing four miles today. It felt great, but didn't push myself.

Took a chance on meals. Double egg patty/sausage between breakfast. Ate some of the macadamia Costco mini cookies and rest of the few sugar free, tiny cookies. Lunch was frozen dinner. Dinner was lobster ravioli (yikes, 1100mg sodium per servings (2 serving). I ate half, felt fine.

Ate the rest of the macadamia cookies, BP rose a little. All things considered, doing pretty well.

Seems like high sodium or high sugars, with high histamines, seems to be the problem. Histamines mostly being the problem.

Bedtime

Proactively took a melatonin at bedtime because of all the sugar I had today.

Also took a small half of a Benadryl. They tend to break slightly unevenly so I take which uneven side seems most useful.

10 July 2022 Sunday

Woke a bit tired with a sinus headache again. Probably should spend day(s) flushing again every hour.

Trying caffeinated tea today. If that doesn't kill me, may try on another day, even with honey(?).

Well...not liking the reaction from the caffeine. Though I had a double/double shot of espresso today, as yesterday. Tea caffeine, not so much fun, apparently.

Sore today. From the four miles yesterday, probably. Feeling old today, but good. Like I got exercise, again! Yay!

Out of sweets now. Just Costco small biscotti left. Ate rest of lobster ravioli to see how the sodium issue lays with me today, slightly larger portion than yesterday's.

I know I've been craving sweets a bit lately, and that can be a symptom of some of the possible conditions I may be experiencing. Or low daily protein intake. But this week I've been craving food in general, even more so. I'm wondering now if it might not be a good sign of increasing better health.

I just need to get more exercise, more normal daily movement. I've been so sick for three months now, that I moved (and wanted to move) very little, to avoid feeling too tired, or more ill. So this may be a good sign. Here's hoping.

Woke hourly, all night. Took no melatonin.

11 July 2022 Monday

Walked three miles, early morning. Would have done four, but it was warming up too so too fast. Tossed out a Costco food/sweet I'd gotten (it was only $3 and I had eaten a bunch already), as it increased my feelings of long covid (sugar and maybe histamine issues). So, I trashed it...took half a Benadryl to help decrease discomfort of feeling of heart beating & high BP.

Used Doordash for the second time, during this free trial month. Then, canceled it. Ordered Yakisoba and some kind of balls of octopus, from Umami Kitchen. Very tasty. Figured I'd cancel on my final day of the trial month, as I'd only used it twice (first time for some very tasty Happy Teriyaki tempura). Decided I needed to get out more and I'd just have to go pick up my own food.

Still waiting to see if what I ate for lunch affects me poorly. So far, so good. Wanted to eat more but thought I'd best wait as a test. Concerned mostly about high sodium issues, maybe histamines also?

Woke hourly through the night, I took no melatonin. Had to relieve myself a lot each time I got up, so that may be what woke me and I just need to moderate my tea drinking at night, so no more waking from it.

12 July 2022 Tuesday

Walked two miles, as I got started late.

9:30AM The sun was beating down. Supposed to be 85 degrees today, again. 84 was high yesterday.

No melatonin at bedtime.

Woke every hour or so to get up and relieve myself. Have to get drinking herbal teas late, under control. I think it's just drinking too much liquid too late into the evening.

13 July 2022 Wednesday

Could feel virus-heart/BP when I woke up. Then dozed for a while and felt better.

Did 5.4 miles today! After the last five mile debacle, this felt great to accomplish. Took half a Benadryl at the start, as I woke feeling a bit weird today. Maybe from the big Ummii Kitchen lunch yesterday, which I kind of expected.

The walk felt good, but left shoulder almost started to ache, both hands were a little swollen, last half mile was getting weird. Drank the rest of my water (I always carry a small bottle in case I need a Benadryl) just as I was making it to the end. I felt worn out, but in a good way.

Took melatonin tonight for good sleep as my VA heart aorta artery ultrasound is tomorrow.

14 July 2022 Thursday

Fasted.

11AM At American Lake Puget Sound VA Hospital for aorta ultrasound down the center of my torso..

Not feeling perfect, having some sinus issues.

Ultrasound completed. All looked good, turned out I hadn't needed to fast at all.

Stopped by Bill's Boathouse on American Lake who came to our high school to teach us and I got certified for SCUBA, in 11th grade, in1971.

It motivated my mom and older sister (by three years), and both got certified that year. But the Boathouse is now gone. It's now just a sad empty lot by the lake, fenced off. I was bummed, but shot video of it on Instagram (account: jzmurdock) and explained what it was. So far I have 30,000+ plays off it.

Stopped by Winco on the way home for groceries.

Got home and had the worst headache, sinus and scalp pain (so also a BP issue, which worried me). Did I catch covid-19 BA5, or something, again? Hospital has very good care about mask use, etc. Damn! I'm so tired of this, all of this.

Took melatonin to (hopefully) assure some sleep.

15 July 2022 Friday

Woke with sinus pain, but sinuses are opened. Just how covid started, too. Then it dropped briefly into my throat for a day (lightly), then into my chest. I'm hoping this time after having contracted it several times, after virus shots, and boosters...maybe it will just dissipate? Hopefully.

9AM Feeling now like long covid may have died off last night.

The sinus pain was its final death throe I (attacking dying animal syndrome). I can now barely feel the virus, slight feeling of vagus nerve irritation. I know covid/LC is a trickster. It feels like it dies, then raises up its hideousness again. So it will probably come back stronger again. Or it's gone another level/step down in its seemingly never ending progress toward dissipation.

One can only and always hope. Going to take it easy today.

I need to straighten up around the house, as I've not felt much like doing it this week/month/past 3 months.

I feel like...a "filth", is missing somewhat from my body/system. I've felt this before over the years with a flu/virus. Someone once told me that a virus makes you ill because you are experiencing its waste product in your system, which is reacting to that. Well, that's disgusting. But that's what it feels like sometimes. When I first heard covid-19 came from bats, what I was feeling in my system felt like that made sense. A virus from a bat would seem to be experienced as a very disgusting, foul feeling, sickening, poisoning.

TODAY IS EITHER A TURNING POINT or, well...not.

Tried the sugar replacement I picked up at Winco (Erythritol, "does not affect blood sugar, so the carbohydrates it contains are considered non-impact"), using it in my tea, half a teaspoon and ate a sugar free cookie.

Had Costco breakfast food (sausage between two egg "patties") for breakfast. Could have less sodium in it but, whatever.

Feeling like that Erythritol evoked stronger feelings of long covid, but only slightly. BP doesn't feel much elevated. So far, so good, but it's not completely gone yet.

12:30PM Just had lunch. My best guess is that I caught a "flavor" of covid yesterday and fought it off. Maybe it helped decrease my LC some, in either the short term or long term? Hopefully, the latter.

Took a melatonin at bedtime.

16 July 2022 Saturday

Woke too early, dozed, woke again feeling heart/BP issues. Turned on "radio" (that is: "Alexa, play KNKX", my local listener-owned radio station that has NPR). Dozed, got up earlier than I wanted, as I was wide awake, anyway.

Feeling the virus more than yesterday, sadly. Had oatmeal with Erythritol, with a banana which is supposed to cause histamine release, but felt pretty good afterward. Still. Not buying bananas again for a while.

Feeling a little something now, virus? BP? Feeling swollen? Something.

I don't think LC is gone, maybe a shift of some sort further toward inactivity?

Took a melatonin to get sleep because of seeing my sister and husband tomorrow evening and waning the best chance for the best sleep I can get.

17 July 2022 Sunday

Woke of course, too early. Dozed to "radio" playing. Virus felt less today, but still there. Feeling... odd today.

Walked three miles. Felt better after, than before.

Seeing my sister & husband this evening for drinks downtown, but I can't drink. Thanks long covid, you suck. Three months, no drinks. No vaping cannabis until three days ago I tested that out. Which I view as progress. Maybe someday (soon?) I can have a glass of wine again.

18 July 2022 Monday

Woke feeling a bit tired. Slept through the night though, getting up only once to relieve myself.

Taking a day off from walking.

To be careful, I checked dosage and one can have up to six Benadryl per day. I've been no where near that and have carefully restricted myself. Took a bit more than normal today, but felt like my body was opening up. I could literally breathe better, esp., through my nostrils. The feeling I've had all day of my "immune system eating itself", has vanished. A good feeling.

Picked up new print getting framed at frame shop and that made me happy.

Felt a bit more viral today, not bad, just annoying.

19 July 2022 Tuesday

Took a morning Valacyclovir.

No melatonin last night. Woke a few times, got back to sleep. Then woke feeling more rested and less viral overall. AM I getting over this? [perhaps, but slowly, verry slowly]

Still feeling a bit of the old vagus nerve condition. Which seems to be lightening up. I'm considering going back on Clariton (loratadine). Had bad effects stopping it cold, earlier this year. Next time I would go off it slowly after having been on it for a while.

Also, going on it takes a few days to acclimate (going to sleep can be hard, or staying asleep at night for a few days). But if it saves my having to take 2-3 Benadryl per day, considering my fears of having to take ever more for the same effect (which hasn't happened yet, but I have concerns and it's best to see these things ahead of time). So, loratadine may be a good, one-a-day option.

Walked only three miles today, as it was getting too warm, even though I started early. I took half a Benadryl at beginning of walk.

Time for my Valacyclovir dose at 9AM pill happened during the walk. So I thought I would stop taking it for now, just to see what happens, while I still have many pills for the next two weeks.

Still considering starting Claritin today.

St. Michael's hospital called. My Zio patch heart monitor data came in and and they reviewed it and my heart is normal. Info should be up on the "mychart" website soon. I'll then send it to VA, or if that doesn't work, notify them so they can request it directly.

Melatonin at bedtime.

20 July 2022 Wednesday

Woke a couple of times, but wasn't a big deal.

Woke feeling pretty good. Not feeling all "virally". My heart, etc., feels a little delicate, but it could be me over-perceiving things.

Supposed to be 85 degrees today so, working out under these new conditions (with no Valacyclovir), wondering if I should go for a walk, or not. If so, I need to leave soon to avoid heat.

Pretty happy so far with my condition, as it feels like progress.

Only walked two miles today as it was already getting hot out and was wearing me out and I didn't want to overdo things. Took no Benadryl though, so that's good.

No melatonin at bed.

21 July 2022 Thursday

Woke not feeling the virus/heart stuff so much, though I did some, when waking up middle of night.

2nd day of no Valacyclovir.

Took a Claritin in morning for testing its use out, for this condition.

Noon. Somehow I'm still off the Valacyclovir, but I don't like the feeling I feel. Vagus nerve is very noticeable, a light throbbing of heart in veins, which seem sensitive. I wonder if this is a new stage of healing now that I'll have to put up with and bear through? IF that's all it is, fine. But I'll be so glad to be over this misery.

I looked up how to numb the vagus nerve and there's not much help that I could find. But it did say to splash cold water on your face. Nope, didn't work. Or ice on the back of your neck. OK, tried that and it worked! That lasted almost a couple of hours. Until, it again returned. But I think that's good news that I'm starting to feel normal.

I can't be sure yet, but minus the vagus nerve/body feeling, I think I feel... normal? Without Valacyclovir.

Tomorrow I will not take Claritin, again. I don't think it's working as I need it to. I will try to go back to Benadryl. as it works better. Then I will forget about switching to Claritin. I just thought if I'm taking something throughout the day, one 24 hour pill would be preferable. Even if not better, as it may be turning out.

6:30PM Trying chamomile tea to see if it helps with the vagus nerve issue.

Melatonin at bedtime.

22 July 2022 Friday

Third day, no Valacyclovir.

Got up once to relieve myself, then slept pretty well, with weird dreams, as is normal lately.

Woke sleepy (from melatonin?). Thing I like about melatonin over sleeping pills is, I can shake off the drowsiness in the morning somewhat easily. Feel fairly rested, no viral feelings, Not much feeling of vagus nerve, though perhaps a tiny bit.

Cream of wheat breakfast, w/teaspoon of Erythritol. And a double/double espresso, which I'm so happy to be back up to.

Bought different sugar free things, ice cream, chocolate, cookies, ate some of each and blood pressure stayed the same. More progress perhaps?

No melatonin.

23 July 2022 Saturday

Fourth day, no Valacyclovir.

Woke feeling good again. Noticing that stupid vagus nerve, just a bit, but it's (maybe) lessening each day! Woke with a sinus headache which could have been from going to Fred Meyer's in East Bremerton, a very diff environment (more industrial area), than here in West Bremerton.

Or it could be the sugar substitute sweets I ate a bunch of yesterday. Typically, eating too many sweets in the evening, can leave me waking with a sinus headache, or a kind of "hangover" feeling, similar to if I had drunk alcohol, but without the more severe repercussions alcohol brings with it. In being after all, a kind of solvent. Sugar, alcohol, affect one's blood sugar or insulin levels. Overusing those things pound on one's insulin receptors until they can shrivel, leading to diabetes. Or obversely abusing one's insulin in other ways that can lead to hypoglycemia, as my ex wife had years ago, until she started on a natural sugar free diet.

Tulsi tea once a day, with refill of hot water for a second cup.

Walked four miles. It felt great by end of three miles, but very ready to be done by end of four miles.

24 July 2022 Sunday

Woke feeling good.

Tested eating lentils for lunch. Felt good, until later when I had to take Benadryl [and woke feeling issues from it on Monday], though doing well. Vagus nerve is slowly healing?

Tulsi tea once a day, refill with hot water, drinking second cup.

No melatonin.

25 July 2022 Monday

Woke too early, turned on "radio", dozed. This is odd for me. All my life I was used to getting up early (4:30AM/5AM), getting right out of bed. I'd heard recently it's not healthy to wake and just lie there for a long time. Best to get up earlier than you want, especially as you get older.

7:30AM Got up, slow to roll out of bed, feeling somewhat lethargic. Some hangover maybe from eating lentils and taking more than normal Benadryl, as I've not used it much these past couple of days. I've noticed all my life on bad allergy/sinus days, overusing antihistamines (and decongestants), can lead one to a kind of hangover the next day. Even though you've solved the previous day's health issues. But doing well now.

Tulsi tea once a day, refill with hot water drinking second cup.

Notified VA doctor about stopping Valacyclovir and about Zio patch, indicating for them to request results as I still can't see it online.

Melatonin.

Chapter 8

26July 2022 Tuesday

Woke early, "radio" on, slept in. Woke, feeling that virus.

Got up, took half a Benadryl after breakfast.

Tulsi tea once a day, refill with hot water drinking second cup. I'm thinking I'm not feeling what I was feeling yesterday. It was nothing I ate (maybe somewhat), but perhaps the virus is returning after stopping the Valacyclovir. We shall see.

Signify called for Aetna to schedule a home doctor visit tomorrow at 5PM toward my Medicare renewal, or something. Standard Medicare service from the supplement insurance company.

What I have here in this virus feeling, is either a lesser state of it after the length of time I've had it, or due to time on Valacyclovir, or it's coming back & eventually to full strength as it was before. And I'll have to go back on Valacyclovir. But as long as it took a while to return, I'm thinking it's lessened in some ways.

Twenty-five sit ups/curls, three sets of eight each of some arm weights [this messed up my back for weeks to come, which I've experienced in recent years when I start lifting weights again, until I get my back strengthened again and then I'm fine. I've gone through this three times before I finally get strengthened enough to not worry about it. Now I'm having problems getting that to work at all]

Melatonin.

27July 2022 Wednesday

Woke feeling pretty good, slight feeling of virus.

Tulsi tea once a day, refill with hot water drinking second cup.

Used elliptical today (I have one in the basement) for 1.5 miles and that beat me down (in a good way) so maybe I'm getting a better workout on that than walking, as it is a various level workout.

Aetna/Signify doctor visit today 5PM was canceled. Nice.

No melatonin.

28 July 2022 Thursday

Sister's 70th birthday. Left her a voicemail as she's in another state, having fun. Good for her! Having retired as a flight attendant, we never know what part of the world she may turn up in.

Had a bad long covid/vagus nerve day, as if it was fighting back before going down to another lower level, toward dissipating (that "attacking dying animal" response). I think (hope). Took a lot of antihistamines today, knocked me out early afternoon in my recliner.

Woke to BP a bit high and pulse racing. Used what VA Nurse said to do, bearing down in my chest muscles, spiking blood pressure and pulse went back down to normal. Generally uncomfortable today. What a life.

Some of the allergy issues today could be from the air conditioner, as that's caused me allergy issues in the past. Air too dry, maybe. Though I do have an air cleaner going. Could also be due to elliptical workout yesterday, to some degree.

Tulsi tea once a day, refill with hot water drinking second cup.

No melatonin.

29 July 2022 Friday

Woke feeling better from LC.

9:30AM Took half a Benadryl. Feeling a bit swollen, maybe due to weather/air conditioner. Supposed to be 92 degrees today. I want to do elliptical today. Woke with sinus issues, but no pain.

Flushed sinuses and felt better, clearing them out some.

Signify/Aetna called today to reschedule and after all their boring phone boilerplate statements, said there's nothing until mid-August [by September, there was still nothing, but they finally called back mid-September for an October appointment]. This is kind of annoying. Whatever...

Walked fifteen minutes on elliptical, about .9 mile. Garage door open and working out feet from it, it was already getting hot, even with a large fan on behind me, and the one on the device going.

Tulsi tea once a day, with second cup.

30 July 2022 Saturday

Woke feeling pretty good.

Tulsi tea once a day, refill with second cup. Let's just accept I'm doing that as a regular thing going forward.

Feeling the vagus nerve issue. I really wish it would just Go Away.

Walked twenty minutes on elliptical, about 1.1 mile. Wanted to do more but it was starting to get hot. 92 degrees today. Felt better in afternoon, esp., early evening.

Melatonin.

31 July 2022 Sunday

Slept well. Woke with sinus headache.

Fell pretty good, maybe a tiny bit better each day. Can feel the virus....vagus nerve, less each day in a "half life" kind of dissipation.

Still...LEAVE FASTER!

No melatonin, trouble getting to sleep, but fine thereafter.

1 August 2022 Monday

Woke feeling, OK.

Switched Vit. C down from 2000/day to 1000mg as the herpes virus activation seems to be fine now with the vagus nerve now as my primary issue.

Felt kind of out of it and unmotivated, today.

2 August 2022 Tuesday

Still just not motivated.

Took melatonin.

3 August 2022 Wednesday

Woke OK, sinuses not great.

Feel like I'm healing some more from long covid.

Until night time, when I don't so much.

Is it coming back? Isn't this getting old?

4 August 2022 Thursday

Son's disenfranchised mother's birthday.

Woke feeling that weird overall body "humming" again of the activated virus. So I started back on 2,000 mg of Vit. C each morning, at least until this film festival I'm in ends on Sunday. I will also be attending an artist friend's exhibition, seventeen miles away in Poulsbo, at 5:30PM tonight.

5 August 2022 Friday

Slept OK, Woke with sinus headache again. Damn if that's not getting old, too. Making me think I caught something at the event last night. Got some walking / exercise done yesterday, which was a trial, pushing through it to make the event yesterday, late afternoon but...I'm feeling better today.

Flushed when I got up, felt better after a bit.

I stopped the anti-virals last week for LC, and I've been feeling good without them. Then went down to 1000 mg of Vit. C per day and... started feeling pretty bad again, yesterday.

But now I'm thinking it's all about having cut back exercise this past week because of the heat.

Still taking the Tulsi tea which seems to be (maybe) helping? Found some Tulsi tea with ginger and turmeric. It's far tastier, so switching to that.

So, WAS it going back to 2000 mg of Vit. C a day again, or lack of exercise? I'm thinking it's both, but mostly the exercise, really.

Lesson learned from this? Do not catch Long covid! Sure, I'll remember that next time...

Obviously.

Ate some chocolate & shortbread cookies today and one keto low sugar ice cream bar, viral reaction was observable, but manageable. As in less than usual. So, progress?

Took Valacyclovir in case that helps with what's going on.

6 August 2022 Saturday

Took Valacyclovir in the morning.

Hit the West Sound Film Festival today at the Historic Roxy Theater downtown Bremerton. Saw festival director Amy, met with people and family and finally got to see my documentary on screen ("Pvt. Ravel's Bolero"). It got a really good applause, the longest up to that point.

Then participated in the on stage Q&A with three other filmmakers for the short documentary block of films. I felt shaky on stage, thought. I hoped I wouldn't fall down or something. But afterward my sister said I presented well and seemed in command of my situation. Even when handed the mic to speak about the making of my film. Shook hands with the filmmaker of the film right after mine, a perfect companion piece to mine. We both seemed very impressed with each other's work.

A couple of hours later, we went down the street to SeeFilm Theater to watch the music video block with the one I worked on ("The Fingers" with The Electric Kühl-Aid Party band with Jack Moriarity (also of "Misery Whip" band), son of cartoonist Pat Moriarty). I filmed some of it, Tyler Darkow filmed some and Kelly Hughes filmed some. He later edited all the footage from the shoot he put together and we watched one of the four songs filmed on this screen. Q&A followed.

We gathered with people for a talk session at the Horse & Cow (a Navy Submariner) bar/restaurant. Sister and husband took off and we moved up to the Roxy Theater and the interview cabana across the street. We were going to get interviewed, myself, Kelly, Tyler and Pat. but I suddenly felt exhausted and not well and had to make my apologies and leave rather abruptly. I had to take Benadryl all day to stay functional.

Still, considering I was on my feet for much of the day, which was quite taxing, I did rather well. It also felt good to go and do something like that again.

Took Valacyclovir in evening.

7 August 2022 Sunday

Woke again with yet another sinus headache. Took a Valacyclovir & flushed a few times. Need to keep flushing hourly to get rid of this. I was after all on the streets of downtown Bremerton all day and around a lot of people for the film festival. Feeling better today, viral load much lowered.

I think after yesterday, feeling the virus humming all through my nerves, I understand a tiny bit what it's like having MS. When I was on stage being interviewed at the film festival about my film, I was hoping I could stand up there until it was over and not fall down. It was a little disturbing and scary. I didn't want to make a big issue falling down on stage.

Today, after Valacyclovir for a couple of days, I am feeling much better. I can't wait until this just goes the hell away! I'm so tired of thinking, saying that. Three miserable months, after two years of this thing off and on, off and on, and this time (last few months) being the WORST, this really quite ENOUGH! Thank you very much!

8 August 2022 Monday

Woke feeling pretty good. Viral load lower. Heart beating too fast, or weirdly. Tried bearing down technique and in a few minutes, it returned to normal.

Last morning of Valacyclovir today for this current issue. Rough day feeling...not bad, but not great.

Took another Valacyclovir in evening, wanting to tamp this damn thing down enough to quit. But when do I quit. And can I? Nuts.

9 August 2022 Tuesday

Woke feeling pretty good.

Took another Valacyclovir in the morning. I do so hate this vagus nerve feeling and being over reactive to food again.

5PM Feeling pretty good.

Took another Valacyclovir & melatonin for hopefully a good night's rest, due to TV interview tomorrow.

10 August 2022 Wednesday

Took a Valacyclovir. Woke with a sinus headache (gee, THAT never happens), took some antihistamines. Which dried me out. NOT great for an on camera interview today at a TV station.

Felt viral/weird all day, which made the interview problematic. Had to drink water before interview and having water on the table during the interview, on BKat TV local channel 12 [see link at end of book for interviews, mine and my friends who were with me]. I didn't want to have to hit the rest room in the middle of being on camera.

My mouth was so dry during the interview. But... it went well and we had a good time. My two friends got interviewed after me. Mine airs in a week. Theirs, two weeks after.

[As of 19 September 2022, mine's aired three times now. Theirs, not at all. As of 22 September 2022, Pat Moriarity's finally aired. Still waiting for Kelly Hughes' interview. Though his and mine are on their YouTube and Vimeo channels. Pat, who had a video on there first, now doesn't have one on YouTube. So odd. You can see these interviews in the links I supplied at the end under, "Personal Links"]

Took another Valacyclovir.

11 August 2022 Thursday

Felt viral again, but not like yesterday. Still, bad.

No Valacyclovir today (yet) but probably need it. And I want to see if I can handle this with Benadryl.

I was hoping that taking a few days of Valacyclovir would lower the viral load enough to return to where I was, so I could stop. I'll know in a day or two. If it comes back and it's too uncomfortable, I'll have to go on a regular daily dose until I run out. Then what?

So...why did I need to go on the Valacyclovir again? Because I over did it at the film festival last weekend. So, if I do too little exercise, I feel ill. Too much? Same result. Sigh...

Using Valacyclovir to normalize me, and a few days to take it easy to heal up. Then I should be back to functional and get back to proper exercise (heat/weather hasn't helped in it being so hot, but I do love the hot weather, normally).

Bedtime, I eventually relented and took a melatonin, as I wasn't getting to sleep for a while.

12 August 2022 Friday

8AM Woke feeling good. Slept in.

Went to see "Top Gun Maverick", at SeeFilm theater. Got "Island Food" on the way home for dinner and got to eat some tasty food. Figured it may be high in things bad for me, but it tasted/felt so good. I took half a Benadryl, as I'm not where I'd like to be. Which is, never again feeling covid/long covid symptoms at all. But probably could have made it without taking anything. So. Progress?

No melatonin.

13 August 2022 Saturday

Slept well, woke a couple of times, but then slept till rested.

Woke feeling a bit of the old virus but...OK.

No melatonin.

14 August 2022 Sunday

Slept pretty good. Woke with no sinus headache, but still not opened up completely and feeling slight virus feeling.

Tried a quarter shot of whiskey today, watered down in a shot glass. Virus seemed to react at first sip, heart beating oddly/heavily, then it seemed to recede. Drank the rest over forty minutes, with no bad effect. It felt good but...I wonder at this point, would alcohol actually speed up the virus dissipating? Where before it would have forced my metabolism to go a bit nuts (high BP spiking)? Curious.

Feeling pretty good this afternoon. Also, curious how I'll feel when I wake up tomorrow.

15 August 2022 Monday

6AM Woke. Feel slight virus, maybe this is a new form of it beginning to fade? This virus has a myriad of ways to decline and feel differently but never dissipate.

Walked 3.4 miles. Felt good.

Had half a pint of Guinness with lunch. Hours later, still feel fine! I drank plenty Guinness & Jameson Whiskey in Ireland in 2015 and walked everywhere, way too much, but had so much fun. And now I can barely do half a pint? Good grief.

Took melatonin.

16 August 2022 Tuesday

Woke feeling slight virus feel. But OK.

Had trouble getting to sleep, did not take melatonin

Got up after falling asleep, took half a Benadryl for viral/histamine heart issue (from lunch most likely), then fell asleep.

17 August 2022 Wednesday

Woke feeling pretty good.

Walked 3.2 miles today and it was getting pretty warm.

Mid afternoon after lunch, ate a pint of sugarfree ice cream & 2 sugar free cookies, two small pieces of sugared chocolate, had an uncomfortable histamine reaction, maybe seeming worse to me now, than it was? As I'm now getting unused to feeling them. Anyway, took an entire Benadryl.

I take it back, it did get rather uncomfortable, but feeling better now.

[a word on sugar replacements. Be careful. Aside from "maybe" causing gas issues in your intestines, new research shows health issues from some. (see ref# 27) For myself I've been trying a blend from Costco of Erythritol and monk fruit sweetener, but I don't use much.]

18 August 2022 Thursday

Woke feeling OK. Took some antihistamines again today.

I think I'm feeling the virus (LC) again. Like I'm needing to take Valacyclovir again. It's not bad, but enough that I'd like to not feel it at all and wondering if a few pills will fend it off. Knock it down. Or if I keep doing this from time to time, I may eventually kill it? Uh huh, and follow me, I have a bridge in Brooklyn I'd like to sell you...

Decided to try Valacyclovir again to see if it changes what I've been feeling, or if it's unnecessary.

19 August 2022 Friday

Woke feeling good. Had trouble sleeping, but finally got to sleep for the biggest part of the night.

Took a Valacyclovir in the morning.

Today took a 3.2 mile walk, took half a Benadryl prior to it. Feeling the virus more today. It was headed up, increasing before Valacyclovir last night. Will a three day course help, or has it become useless? Getting low on Valacyclovir.

Found this from an NPR article:

Post-COVID Syndrome Treatment

> https://www.houstonmethodist.org/global/why-choose-houston-methodist/blog/2020/nov/post-covid-syndrome-what-should-you-do-if-you-have-lingering-covid-19-symptoms/

And, Reduced Myocardial Blood Flow is New Clue in How COVID-19 is Impacting the Heart

> https://www.houstonmethodist.org/newsroom/reduced-myocardial-blood-flow-is-new-clue-in-how-covid-19-is-impacting-the-heart/

20 August 2022 Saturday

5AM Woke from somewhat restless sleep. Felt fairly rested in morning, though.

Feeling the LC virus and don't want to feel it, but very ready for it to DIE!

Feeling my heart some, and it's annoying! And unwelcome. What evoked this change? That I was off antihistamines and now need them again? I think I'm starting to feel better and did need the Valacyclovir.

Is this however just the long covid recycle process again? That I'm not getting better but just headed into another cycle of it? It seems it's been morphing, changing (evolving?), in my having to take Benadryl again. When it was unnecessary (but only for a few days perhaps?).

Damn this is an exhausting disease! It's like it plays mind games on you, over and over and over...

21 August 2022 Sunday

Took my last Valacyclovir of a three day run.

Walked 3 miles (3 mile walks from home are always actually 3.2 miles).

3:30PM Got a body rush, heart beating harder, faster for no reason. It scared me at first, then I remembered... in taking a new course of Valacyclovir, about the time I stop taking it, it's working, as the virus fights back, just before it caves in ("attacking dying animal syndrome"). Hoping it's just that, as my first thoughts were to unlock the front door, in case I have to call 911 but couldn't make it to the door when they arrive. That thought is always there in my considering calling 911. It's just best to be proactive/prepared. And I don't want anyone breaking in my front door). I've had to have this thought way too many times these past few months.

Seven more days until long covid, for this go around (with onset on March 28th) will have been five months.

About five minutes after onset of heart beating hard/fast, it's went back to normal. Well, that was miserably disturbing for a few minutes...

Took a melatonin after not getting to sleep for too long.

22 August 2022 Monday

Woke feeling the virus. What IS going ON?

How much I hate this disease. Took half a Benadryl & half a Chlor. Maleate for my sinuses.

I lied in bed last night wondering if the Costco two egg patties with sausage between breakfast thing I keep around, which I ate for dinner two nights in a row, are what's causing me histamine issues.

So no more until I clear them and test them again.

Yesterday early evening, I felt goodness washing over me. I was feeling better and... my sinuses opened up! This disease seems to affect my sinuses and not just overall body illness feeling, as it hummed along, coursing through my veins.

I've always had sinus issues, but ever since packing B-52 bomber drag chutes in the USAF for years, nearly every day in a closed room with the JP-4 jet fuel exhaust that they're coated with. It filled the air, as I labored to get those forty-eight ribbon panels ordered up and slide into the deployment bag. Then literally repeatedly jumping up and down on it to fit it into its tight bag, And I've seemed ever since to have even worse sinus and allergy issues all through my life.

Jet fuel has heavy metals and toxic chemicals in it. So how does the exhaust not have remnants of that remaining? I'm still considering seeking disability, as one of my VA doctors told me to do. He said even if I only received a 10% disability for it, that may become more important as I get older.

I should go on a walk today, But I just don't feel like it. It's heating up outside. Low 80s today supposedly, and I have to go to Silverdale to pick up a print job of my film poster (from "Pvt. Ravel's Bolero"), and Kelly's poster for our "The Fingers" music video we both worked on. Both posters were up at the recent West Sound Film Festival. I later picked them up from the Historic Roxy Theater, where the festival was held in part. I had requested them of the festival director since they made them up for all the shown Official Selection films and would just dispose of them anyway.

Surprising (to me) UPDATE on results of my taking Valacyclovir:

June 28, after stopping the meds it took three weeks before I felt I needed to go back on the meds.

July 19, after stopping the meds it took two weeks before I felt I needed to go back on the meds.

August 5-11, after stopping the meds, it took one week before I felt I needed to go back on the meds.

August 18-21, I needed them again.

===========

EMAIL composed, but not sent to VA doctor:

Hi,
This is an update & request.
First, the reason I'm a pain in the neck about my long covid situation is I'm a

systems analyst, author & filmmaker I dig into things. I have a university degree in psychology/phenomenology, perfect for observing something like I'm going through.

I took the prescribed thirty day supply of Valacyclovir and tried to use it as little as possible.

I've also been eating & exercising, no alcohol (this disease forces you to be healthier it seems), all which helped. I've been eating low histamine foods & no sugar, two things that exacerbate this condition, spiking Blood Pressure & Heart Rate (mostly BP).

What I've found surprised me, regarding my schedule of use of Valacyclovir:

June 28, stopped Valacyclovir after being on it for a while. Then,

3 weeks, no Valacyclovir until I needed it again. Then,

3 days, taking Valacyclovir ending July 19. Then,

2 weeks, without Valacyclovir. Then,

August 11, first day of no Valacyclovir. Then,

1 week no Valacyclovir. before needing it again. Then,

August 18-21, on Valacyclovir. Then,

August 22, feeling a bit rough already.

What I've come to believe from this data is that long use of it works well (3 weeks before needing it again).

But taking it sporadically only when I need it, decreases those periods (from 3 weeks, to 2 weeks, to 1 week), a starkly obvious result.

That might say to some that it's working less. What it says to me is that I need to be on it long term.

I'll be 67 on the 30th of August 2022, and it would be nice to feel better, than worse that day.

All that being said, could I get another, at least thirty day supply, holding me over until my teleMed appointment with the doctor. and we can go from there?

That's all I have.

Thanks.

23 August 2022 Tuesday

Woke with heart flutters. Damn. Then fell back asleep, laid in bed for a bit and had the heart issue for a long time (maybe hours?).

Got up after trouble getting back to sleep and took half a Benadryl, which eventually helped.

Walked 3 miles today, and before the last half mile, took a half Benadryl.

Chapter 8

Composed version of email (above) I finally sent:

Hi,
I took the doctor's thirty day supply of Valacyclovir and tried to use it as little as possible. I really didn't want to just take it straight through, then run out and be stuck without, and miserable.
I've been eating & exercising, no alcohol (this disease forces you to be healthier, it seems), all which helps. I've been eating low histamine foods & no sugar, two things that exacerbate this condition, spiking blood pressure &/or heart rate (mostly BP).
What I've found surprised me regarding my schedule of use of Valacyclovir:
June 28 stopped Valacyclovir after being on it for a while (2 weeks?). Then,
3 weeks of no Valacyclovir until I felt I really needed it again. Then,
3 days of Valacyclovir ending July 19. Then,
2 weeks without Valacyclovir. Then,
August 11 first day no Valacyclovir. Then,
1 week no Valacyclovir. before needing it again then
August 18-21 on Valacyclovir.
August 22, feeling a bit rough already.
What I've come to believe from this data is that extended use of Valacyclovir works well (3 weeks before needing it again). But taking Valacyclovir sporadically only when I need it, decreased the periods (from 3 weeks, to 2 weeks, to 1 week), a starkly obvious result.
That might say to some it's working less. What it says to me though is I need to be on it longer term.
I'll be 67 on the 30th of August and it would be nice to feel better than worse on that day.
So, could I get another thirty day supply, to hold me over until my teleMed appt with the doctor and we can go from there? If I don't need it, I won't take it, but I'd like to have it if I need it, as its cyclical nature can confuse things. I do feel I'm getting stronger/healthier. I also can't help but wonder if being on it is helping me get over it more quickly.
That's all I have.
Thanks for your time.

24 August 2022 Wednesday

I've been feeling the long covid very lightly today, a good feeling.

As a another test, I ate a sugarless cookie, a sugarless peanut butter cup and another sugarless cookie. I'm feeling LC more in my heart beating (BP) harder (not faster), but still not that much. Is this a low part of the cycle? Will tomorrow bring more, not less? Probably either the cookies or the chocolate PB cup, sugarless or not, are causing this.

8PM I'm feeling pretty good now.

Trouble sleeping, took a melatonin.

25 August 2022 Thursday

Woke too early (4AM), dozed for a few hours.

Took 1/2 a Benadryl in the morning.

Took a melatonin at bedtime, knowing I'd have trouble after this few days of no exercise.

26 August 2022 Friday

Woke about every hour, all night until the last few.

Walked four miles today, and it felt great!

Long covid feels like it's waning and I can only hope. Because that's all it allows us.

27 August 2022 Saturday

Not a great sleep last night, kept waking up. Not as bad as the night before, but took no melatonin last night.

Woke a bit tired, but not feeling virus a lot. Until breakfast, then somewhat.

Took melatonin at bedtime.

28 August 2022 Sunday

Woke a few times. Why has this been happening lately?

Walked three miles, started a fourth but decided three was plenty for today.

Took an evening Valacyclovir because of my birthday coming up. I have five pills left.

29 August 2022 Monday

Miserable sleep AGAIN last night. Woke WAY too early and... after the smoke alarm went off at 4AM! Then a few minutes later! Then a few hours later! No smoke. [some might think I need to change the battery. In the next few weeks, I changed that battery multiple times...I'm thinking there's something wrong with the device]

8AM Tired. Took Valacyclovir. Birthday dinner today with my sister and husband.

5:30PM Dinner at Boat Shed restaurant on the dock. Beautiful evening. We had a great time. Until leaving, Joe drove one way the wrong way up a nearby street. He got annoyed looks, but all was fine. After I moved here, I also drove the wrong way up that same street the first time.

8PM Took Valacyclovir

30 August 2022 Tuesday

Birthday! Spent the day munching on tasting things (too much, but hey, it's my birthday and there's little else to do, other than...) watched a bunch of fun movies. My late mother was born on my birthday. I used to tease her about this. First time I said that, she looked at me, asking how is that possible? I said, "Well God planned for me, so..." And she just smiled and said, "Oh, honey, you weren't planned." We both laughed.

I had a good day, overall. I could have felt better, but I'm quite happy, overall.

Took last of my Valacyclovir in the evening.

Took melatonin at bed.

31 August 2022 Wednesday

Slept well. Woke up a bit burned out, maybe from what I ate yesterday, in partying for my birthday but, it was worth it!

Feeling like I'm still having allergy issues. It's just hard to tell with this condition.

Started working on this book, on Long covid.

1 September 2022 Thursday

Slept well, woke early. Turned "radio" on, dozed for a while longer.

Felt less "viral" today. I think the zinc I started yesterday is helping. Curious how the pantothenic acid might work out once I pick some up.

Took 2 zinc today

Ordered pantothenic acid, should arrive Saturday. I could not find any in local stores. I only want 300mg tabs but there's 250mg and 500mg. [I thought I'd ordered 250mg, but when it arrived I had ordered 500mg tabs. Since I got LC, that kind of mistake hasn't been that unusual.]

2 September 2022 Friday

Slept well. Woke feeling the virus a bit. Took 1 zinc today.

I'm feeling BP a bit high and wondering if it's the zinc. I'm going to stop it to see what happens.

3 September 2022 Saturday

Took zinc with vitamins at breakfast. Slept OK. Feeling less virus than yesterday morning.

My question is, if zinc is making me feel the virus, is it exacerbating it, or is the virus just showing itself more as it is being put down by the zinc ("attacking dying animal syndrome" again)?

Or was yesterday unrelated to the zinc? More of the same with this LC.

Pantothenic acid supplements should arrive today. A little nervous about taking it as I've had poor reactions to some other supplements during covid sensitivity that were intense to some things. Like the Krill oil, when I thought I might be dying. That was pretty horrific. IF it was the Krill oil, or covid making me sensitive or allergic to it. [as of 27 September 2022, still haven't tried either the Pantothenic acid, or the GABA I picked up at my brother's suggestion, to help with sleep rather than using melatonin]

Walked three miles and would have done more except for my left ankle hurting, that I've been trying to heal up using cannabis salve, and also, alternately using heat and cold. [stopped using the cannabis salve as I was perhaps using it too much, bought some "Biofreeze" gel with menthol]. Another day or two and it may get there. [27 September 2022 and it's finally starting to feel better]

Took half a Benadryl when I got home.

Took a shower.

11AM Heart is beating too strongly (high BP) in my chest & neck. So I took another half Benadryl...but is zinc doing this? I started taking zinc and now I'm feeling this issue again which I hadn't been for a while. So...maybe?

Got an email saying that the request I sent my VA doctor asking for another thirty day supply of valocycliver was now in process and I should have it by Thursday. I'd asked for it a week before my birthday so I'd have it before that day (which was five days ago), so it would be active on my birthday. Well. I had some anyway that I used for this (always have a backup plan if you can...always have a "plan b" (and a "plan c" and a "plan d"...)).

This will be helpful to see if I need it. Taking it again to see if it does anything. Or have it on hand if LC recycles back on.

4 September 2022 Sunday

Slept well. Woke feeling the virus, only slightly.

Sinus issues less, but still there. Seasonal allergies perhaps, though it's interesting when I'm on valocycliver for a while, my sinus issues feel prominently relieved.

I just hope I don't get locked into this condition, and one day can get back to what I consider, normal.

5 September 2022 Monday Labor Day

Hope everyone had a great Labor Day holiday!

Slept well. Woke but laid in bed for a long while. Summer is nearly over...

I feel the virus, but it's fuzzy, as if in the final stages. Not the electric buzzing it once was (damn I hated that and the Valacyclovir really helped with it).

6 September 2022 Tuesday

Woke feeling a light version of the virus. Lied in bed a long time listening to the "radio".

By time I got up, I didn't feel the virus so much. After a while, I took a Benadryl anyway.

Received Valacyclovir today! Thought I'd wait until after... IF, I get the new updated booster.

Went to Safeway who said they'll have Pfizer booster Friday, but you have to make an online appointment. Got home, took a Valacyclovir. Thought I'd take it for at least three days, stop, then get a booster on Monday. Maybe.

Friday, I'll make an appointment for a booster shot.

This is interesting, five hours after taking a Valacyclovir my sinuses started feeling better. There was a kind of relaxation, and then they just felt better.

8PM Valacyclovir.

My son, who manages a health food store and sells CBD products, pointed out that the cannabis salve I was using for my strained ankle, might have something to do with some of the odd feelings I've been experiencing. So what I've been feeling may not be LC. So I stopped using it to see what happens.

Took a melatonin as in starting Valacyclovir, it goes better that way.

7 September 2022 Wednesday

Valacyclovir 8AM. Felt a bit fuzzy (virally, not a big deal, just annoying), lied in bed for a long time. Got up feeling pretty good though, but looking forward to positive changes from the Valacyclovir in a few days.

Received GABA supplement today, to help with sleeping. I'll test it along with the Panthothenic acid.

After the past five months, I'm very leery trying anything new.

Walked FOUR miles today, it's taken a while to get back up to that. Ankle felt good (icing and applying heat), overall feel good.

Took some more Benadryl, thinking taking Valacyclovir makes LC want to fight back, so feeling more heart (BP?) issues.

8 September 2022 Thursday

Woke a bit early buy feeling pretty good. Listened to "radio" as I dozed. Then got up, earlier than I have been this week (adjusting to being on Valacyclovir again maybe?).

Had a nice lunch, drank my first full pint of Guinness in over six months. Been having some light BP issues I think, from starting the Valacyclovir?

 If this works like last time, a few more days and the LC should flare up, then go away. Here's hoping.

I should take a melatonin tonight.

9 September 2022 Friday

I slept through the night and woke up briefly twice, feeling a headache, that I think was blood pressure. Turned on NPR. Dozed in bed. Woke up finally, listened to the news for a few minutes and got up. I took half a Chlorpheniramine maleate. Saline flushed my sinuses. Ate a protein breakfast (sausage with two egg patties from Costco), then went for a walk.

Supposed to get up to the 80s today and there's a smoke warning for forest fires, somewhere. I'm feeling the virus, as I like to say when I can feel my heart beating high up in my chest and lower in my throat, a bit. Which I'm assuming is from the Valacyclovir irritated virus.

I made an appointment at Safeway for 1PM Monday to get the updated Pfizer booster shot. I will stop taking the Valacyclovir Saturday morning, as I saw from a 2021 recommendation to stop it at least one day before getting a COVID-19 shot (and another indicating it doesn't matter at all). So I'll add one day to that to be sure, since I couldn't find any new, or 2022 updated information. Always err on the side of caution when possible.

I'm feeling pretty good today, but also feeling a little bit rough. Possibly from drinking (only, but...) a full pint of Guinness yesterday, and eating some other foods, trying to push my limits a little bit. Basically trying to get to acting normal to see how it affects me.

Last night it wasn't affecting me very well. So I took one and a half Benadryl over the early evening, which helped a lot. But as I hadn't been having to, before I started the Valacyclovir again… I'm assuming a slight flareup of the virus from that, is a good sign.

I do expect that once I'm on Valacyclovir for a while, again, sometime after I get the booster shot on Monday, I will start back on it again, and that at some point LC will flare up a bit. Then dissipate. Until I stop Valacyclovir again and I am off it for a while. Then it will probably slowly start to ebb back over time. Or not. As I've said... just go AWAY!

I walked four miles two days ago, and felt great. I got to the end of three miles today and went for the fourth mile because it felt so good. Feels great to be outside, and I guess the endorphin rush added to that. It felt incredible to be at a point where I would feel that feeling. I'm hoping now, that four miles will be my default and I'm done with three mile walks. I'd love to get up to a five mile walks, several times each week, which should be enough for each day. I read somewhere that for normal people at least two fives mile walks per week was healthy.

Forest fires in Washington state alert was received on my Alexa Show, regarding the weekend.

10 September 2022 Saturday

Smoke alert for Bremerton received. Last time this happened a year ago (which was the worst I've ever seen here), even with my air cleaner on high I still had bad allergy problems.

11 September 2022 Sunday

Woke several times, feeling a little uncomfortable with my heart beating, as it was very noticeable. Got up to relieve myself again at 2:30AM and took half a Benadryl. Then slept through the night.

Woke in the morning feeling not too bad.

Forest fire alerts. So canceling my walk today and rather sad about it. A little hazy outside in the early morning.

After breakfast, feeling heart beating a lot (noticeable in my chest and throat), wondering if this is an allergy issue from the air quality, exacerbating LC, so I took half a Benardyl. [I'm not sure that was the case]

Gorst Underground Film Festival film blocks day, was to be today (I was a cofounder with Kelly Hughes, some years back, though I've had to back off these past two years to adviser level, due to LC). This was to be a limited version festival day, no films, just vendors and bands, as our venue was canceled on us at the last minute for this past Friday/Saturday.

Got to go to the event for about an hour, but the high level of forest fire smoke yesterday and today affected me negatively. My heart started to pound, not too bad, but indicative of it not being good being out and since official statement saif that if you're sensitive, don't go out, I probably should (and did) go home.

Had a good day. Off the Valacyclovir, and pretty much, I'm feeling not too bad.

12 September 2022 Monday

Woke feeling OK, though feeling a soft/cottony, viral feeling that went mostly away after getting up and eating.

Today is the updated Pfizer booster shot at 1PM at Safeway.

Got the shot. Feeling nothing, yet.

Wouldn't it be nice...if it killed this LC?

I will have to wait until tomorrow to see, though the virus...the heart beating issue is less. But then the next day is more uncomfortable than the first day, and the day after that even more so, typically. So I'll know in a couple of days.

At bedtime, so far happy with the result of the shot. [that's about to change]

13 September 2022 Tuesday

I woke at 2:30AM with a blood pressure headache, which disturbed me. I relaxed the muscles in the top of my head (scalp) and amazingly, the headache eased. Updated Booster shot issue? I don't think so, this has actually been cropping up slightly over the past week.

[At my next teleMed meeting with my doctor on Friday, he says this is an anxiety issue disconnect from the symptomatic system, exhibiting symptoms of anxiety disconnected from any mental state or reason for it and this is an issue for some people. I hope not. Or is it just another gift from LC that may one day go away also?]

I woke at 3:30AM, fell back asleep. Again at 4:30AM and dozed until I got up at 5:39AM, not feeling that annoying vagus nerve LC feeling. As if, it had gone away. NO, I do not trust that is the case. Did the updated booster yesterday help me, eradicate LC? I can only hope, but still can not trust that. Just wishful thinking.

I feel very slight soreness at vaccine site, but no big deal. Other than that, not experiencing anything bad from shot. Yet.

Ate a couple of sweets to see what happened. Heart beat issues came up so I took a Benadryl. Not over this thing yet, then.

I'm feeling that overall fuzzy feeling that requires Valacyclovir, but want to wait a few days if possible due to the booster shot yesterday. I don't think it matters really, but wanted to try to hold off, anyway. I found an article from the British Herpes Viruses Association (see ref# 28) saying acyclovir/Valacyclovir are specifically targeting the herpes virus, so you can take it without it affecting the covid-19 virus / booster shots.

14 September 2022 Wednesday

Woke not feeling the virus or heart/BP issues. I do seem to be sleeping better this week.

Got up, ate breakfast (oatmeal, & espresso) and only then felt a bit of the heart issues, but seemingly slighter each day since Monday's updated booster shot. I wish I could jump ahead a week and see how I'm feeling then. [OK, two weeks later 27 September 2022, I'm feeling better than before I got the shot, but definitely some discomfort in between and during that week post booster shot]

Most of the day, I'm not feeling that well. Not bad, just not great. Feeling the vagus nerve more than usual lately. Took a half Benadryl.

Feeling better after dinner. Eating seems to have a lot to do with feeling better, when I wait too long to eat, I can go downhill.

Didn't feel great Virus/BP wise, feeling heart beating way too much.

I'm thinking it was all the pepperoni on the pizza. I'd read dried fish or meats have high histamines. I'd eaten this same frozen pizza brand last time and I don't remember any issues. So probably the pepperoni I'd added (always do with frozen home pizza, you have to as they seldom supply much meat. Or, could have been the booster shot. Maybe both.

15 September 2022 Thursday

Slept well (again). Woke early, felt a blood clotting issue in my right inner calf vein where I'd had issues before, and in my upper forehead. I believe it is at or near the branch in my leg, splitting the anterior tibial artery with the peroneal artery. I just read someone in a social media LC group mention healthcare providers seem completely ignorant of micro (blood) clots. Interesting. Maybe? Maybe not.

Had sinus headache that felt a little like a blood pressure issue. But the weather changed, it was cooler this morning which typically gives me sinus issues. Considered taking an 81mg aspirin but fell asleep. Woke an hour later, headache there, but not the clotting issue feeling. So I got up.

Feeling better than last night, but have a weirder virus "ill" feeling overall. I figure some of this is the Monday booster, in my assimilating it, or something.

Felt better around lunch time and after eating some food.

Took a small aspirin after dinner.

Flushing my sinuses today helped.

16 September 2022 Friday

Woke with high blood pressure & a headache. Relaxed myself and felt the headache ease. I think this is a combination of the booster shot on Monday messing with my system & LC. And, summer coming to an end, with the weather changing and it's getting cooler out. Not to mention, today is the first day in a week that the air quality was normal, without forest fire smoke.

TeleMed appt with VA Doctor went very well.

We went over my tests from this past year, all of which said I'm healthy (except for LC which doesn't seem to show up anywhere). Some of the waking-with-BP issues/headache seems to be anxiety issues (as mentioned above, which are not mental/emotional). So we'll go from here to see how it goes. I expect to get better through next week, related to this week's condition being perhaps (probably) due to the booster shot. We set a year from now for my next annual appointment. [VA called a week later to set up an appointment for May 2023 as that's a year from my last annual appointment]

Took a small aspirin with dinner due to the weird sinus headache that may be in part due to blood clotting issues. Did I catch covid again?

My health this week from the poor smokey air quality and my reaction to the covid updated booster shot, has stopped my working on this book now, for several days.

Final log entry day for this Long Covid book?

17 September 2022 Saturday

Nope.

Woke with a weirdly bad sinus headache, that almost didn't feel like sinus issues. LC does keep you guessing, and guessing.

After breakfast, it faded, Flushed sinuses, and sinus headache faded. I took a home covid test, which came up negative. That was a relief.

By noon after lunch, I felt like covid was nearly gone. I can only hope.

Drove to my kid's spouses' family's dinner in Tacoma at Ruston Point, at the Wild Fin restaurant at the beautiful Puget Sound/Commencement Bay waterfront. Instagrammed a video, crossing the bridge (and another at night on the way home). Beautiful down there.

It was colder than I'd expected and I didn't bring a jacket and it was making me feel worse. I wasn't feeling too well. Walked around, lots of people about, not feeling very well for about half an hour. Smelled lots of cannabis vapers having at it. But a very family atmosphere with all happy people having fun.

Great birthday dinner party, a good time. Once seated, I felt better and had a fun time. Furthest and latest I've been out since I got this version of covid/LC over six months ago.

The drive home was actually enjoyable. I got video again, this time while going across the original Narrows Bridge, on Instagram. Felt exhausted when I got home, so I went to bed.

18 September 2022 Sunday

Woke a couple of times too early, then slept through. Woke feeling good, but still a bit tired. Turned on the "radio", dozed. Then finally got up and still felt good.

Oatmeal & espresso for breakfast.

Walked 4 miles and it felt great.

I still feel a little underlying feel of the virus all over, but fairly minimal.

Nice day, sun is out today. 73 degrees at 10:30AM.

Had last night's dinner leftovers for lunch (Parmesan encrusted sole and polenta)...so tasty.

19 September 2022 Monday

Woke feeling pretty good. Slightly too cool nights, warm days now. I'll take the warm days.

By afternoon, I felt the activated virus a bit too much again, to the point that I took a Valacyclovir at 4PM, realizing that it does seem to be making a comeback. And so it goes...

So what do I do now? I do think as time has passed, and compared to my first LC experience which went away over early 2021, that this too is on it's way away. Maybe I'll go back on the Valacyclovir for a while, longer than just three days, or not. I'll have to judge that along the way.

But keeping the viral load low as it dissipates, can't hurt. Unless it proves to not work that way. At which time I still stop taking it. It's a kind of game, or puzzle one has to go along with, to work out and hopefully bring to a conclusion. Or it may just go away regardless on its own. Time will tell, hopefully sooner than later.

And with that, I'll end my daily logs here...

Odds & Ends

From a UC Davis .edu article (link at below):

Some long-haulers show improvements after getting the vaccine

Early data suggested that vaccines provided relief for many long-haulers, but 10 to 15% said they felt worse after getting them. At UC Davis Health, the results have been more positive. According to Sandrock, many patients said they felt better after getting the covid-19 vaccine. "Not one I've seen said they felt worse after getting the covid vaccine. There had been a concern that by getting the vaccine, their symptoms might get worse, but we haven't seen it," Sandrock said.

The reactivation of a previous virus may be causing long covid symptoms

A study published in the journal Cell found reactivation of the Epstein-Barr Virus (EBV) to be a factor in developing long covid. EBV is the virus that causes mononucleosis. The virus is also associated with chronic fatigue syndrome, which resembles long covid symptoms for some people. According to Nam Tran, a professor of clinical pathology, the usual screening test for EBV, known as a heterophile antibody test, is not appropriate for evaluating EBV reactivation. But there are other serology tests — blood tests —that are. One EBV serology test looks at four different markers to determine if the infection is acute, recent, past or a reactivation. Another test looks at the EBV viral load and may be preferred over serology when evaluating reactivation cases. "The EBV serology or EBV viral load test can reveal if reactivation may be contributing to some symptoms experienced by long covid patients," Tran said.

CORONAVIRUS February 11, 2022

11 things doctors have learned about long covid (see, ref# 29)

https://health.ucdavis.edu/news/headlines/11-things-doctors-have-learned-about-long-haul-CoViD/2022/02

Chapter 9

Reference / Research URL Links

1 – NPR - Study finds long COVID can affect your ability to exercise

https://www.npr.org/2022/10/16/1129355122/study-finds-long-covid-can-affect-your-ability-to-exercise

2 – Mayo Clinic - Coronavirus disease 2019 (COVID-19)

https://www.mayoclinic.org/diseases-conditions/coronavirus/symptoms-causes/syc-20479963

3 - Ending Isolation and Precautions for People with COVID-19: Interim Guidance - CDC

https://www.cdc.gov/coronavirus/2019-ncov/hcp/duration-isolation.html

4 - Cytokine Storm

https://www.nejm.org/doi/full/10.1056/NEJMra2026131#:~:text=Cytokine%20storm%20and%20cytokine%20release,autoimmune%20conditions%2C%20and%20%20monogenic%20disorders

5 – NIH - Phenomenological Approaches in Psychology and Health Sciences

https://www.ncbi.nlm.nih.gov/pmc/articles/PMC3627202/

6 - Scientific Breakthrough Against COVID-19: Antibodies Identified That May Make Coronavirus Vaccines Unnecessary

https://scitechdaily.com/scientific-breakthrough-against-covid-19-antibodies-identified-that-may-make-coronavirus-vaccines-unnecessary/

7 - Reduced Myocardial Blood Flow Is New Clue In How Covid-19 Is Impacting The Heart

https://www.houstonmethodist.org/newsroom/reduced-myocardial-blood-flow-is-new-clue-in-how-CoViD-19-is-impacting-the-heart/

8 - UCLA researchers discover how the body regenerates blood vessel lining -

Findings could lead to new methods to help prevent clots and repair damage linked to stents (2018) https://newsroom.ucla.edu/releases/ucla-researchers-discover-how-the-body-regenerates-blood-vessel-lining

9 - Veterans Health Administration (VHA) Coronavirus Disease 2019 (COVID-19) Response Report - Annex B December 15, 2021

https://www.va.gov/health/docs/VHA-COVID-19-Response-2021-Annex-B.pdf

10 – USPSTF Aspirin Use to Prevent Cardiovascular Disease: Preventive Medication

https://www.uspreventiveservicestaskforce.org/uspstf/recommendation/aspirin-to-prevent-cardiovascular-disease-preventive-medication

11 - COVID-19 is a systemic vascular hemopathy: insight for mechanistic and clinical aspects -

[This one in particular I found disturbing] - In the affected microcirculation, innumerable intraluminal pillars (circles), seen as small holes in the cast, reflect the process of intussusceptive angiogenesis (bar = 100um)

https://link.springer.com/article/10.1007/s10456-021-09805-6

12 - Attention deficit/hyperactivity disorder (ADHD) is associated with altered heart rate asymmetry

https://pubmed.ncbi.nlm.nih.gov/25669682/#:~:text=Attention%20deficit%2Fhyperactivity%20disorder%20

13 - Department of Health - Exposure to Smoke from Fires

https://health.ny.gov/environmental/outdoors/air/smoke_from_fire.htm#:~:text=Smoke%20can%20contain%20many%20different,%2C%20styrene%2C%20metals%20and%20dioxins

14 - Is Chicken Soup Really Good for the Common Cold? - McGill, Office for Science and Society, "Separating Sense from Nonsense"

https://www.mcgill.ca/oss/article/food-health-you-asked/there-really-something-story-chicken-soup-good-common-cold#:~:text=Modern%20research%20has%20actually%20shown,such%20as%20pepper%20and%20garlic

15 - What Does COVID Do to Your Blood?

https://www.hopkinsmedicine.org/health/conditions-and-diseases/coronavirus/what-does-covid-do-to-your-blood

16 - Long COVID Symptoms Linked to Effects on Vagus Nerve

https://www.webmd.com/lung/news/20220215/covid-symptoms-linked-to-vagus-

<u>nerve</u>

17 - Longer-term Effects of COVID-19 Infection on Blood Vessels And Blood pressure (LOCHINVAR) (LOCHINVAR) – Very interesting article.

https://clinicaltrials.gov/ct2/show/NCT05087290

Preliminary results showed that participants who had COVID-19 infection had an 8.6mmHg increase in their average 24hr systolic blood pressure, compared to those that did not have COVID-19 infection.

18 - Post Acute Coronavirus (COVID-19) Syndrome

https://www.ncbi.nlm.nih.gov/books/NBK570608/

19 - How to Spot Fake News: Triangulation for Communications Pros

https://spinsucks.com/communication/how-to-spot-fake-news/

20 - Blood abnormalities found in people with Long Covid

Study implicates lack of key hormone, battle-weary immune cells, and reawakened viruses

https://www.science.org/content/article/blood-abnormalities-found-people-long-covid

21 - C.A.R.E. for Long COVID Act (Comprehensive Access to Resources and Education)

https://www.survivorcorps.com/advocacy

22 - Long covid and the Americans with Disabilities Act

https://askjan.org/blogs/jan/2021/03/Long-CoViD-and-the-Americans-with-Disabilities-Act.cfm

23 - Why vitamin C won't 'boost' your immune system against the coronavirus

https://www.livescience.com/coronavirus-vitamin-c-myth.html

24 - Antivirals in the time of COVID-19 – not as easy as it looks!

"Acyclovir is a direct action antiviral. After having been phosphorylated in triphosphate acyclovir by a viral thymidine-kinase only present in virus-infected cells, it acts as a selective competitive inhibitor of the viral polymerase DNA. The incorporation of this nucleoside analogue stops the DNA chain's elongation, thus interrupting the synthesis of viral DNA. Viral replication is thus blocked.

"This method can also be used against HSVs and VZVs.
"Other herpes medications are: Valacyclovir, which is merely an acyclovir prodrug and brings with it much improved bioavailability with oral administration. There is also famciclovir."

https://www.ncbi.nlm.nih.gov/pmc/articles/PMC7560379/

25.- Varicella-zoster virus reactivation causing herpes zoster ophthalmicus (HZO) after SARS-CoV-2 vaccination – report of three cases -

"A 72-year-old woman with no history of autoimmune pathology, candidate for cataract surgery, presented 13 days after the first dose of a Moderna mRNA vaccine with an eruption in the left V1 dermatome. All patients presented the VZV infection after their first dose of a mRNA type of vaccine. Treatment with Valacyclovir 1000 mg × 3/ day for 7–14 days was efficient in all cases."

https://www.ncbi.nlm.nih.gov/pmc/articles/PMC8443850/

26 - Long-Term Administration of Valacyclovir Reduces the Number of Epstein-Barr Virus (EBV) - I infected B Cells but Not the Number of EBV DNA Copies per B Cell in Healthy Volunteers -

"Valacyclovir reduces the frequency of EBV-infected B cells when administered over a long period and, in theory, might allow eradication of EBV from the body if reinfection does not occur."

https://www.ncbi.nlm.nih.gov/pmc/articles/PMC2772668/#:~:text=Valacyclovir %20reduces%20the%20frequency%20of,if%20reinfection%20does%20not %20occur

27 - The unusual relationship between COVID-19 and blood pressure

https://whyy.org/articles/the-unusual-relationship-between-covid-19-and-blood-pressure/

**28 - Valacyclovir therapy and COVID-19 messenger RNA vaccination -
"In summary, I would not delay the COVID-19 mRNA vaccine but administer as scheduled, one day after completion of the Valacyclovir therapy."**

https://www.aaaai.org/allergist-resources/ask-the-expert/answers/old-ask-the-experts/Valacyclovir

29 - 11 things doctors have learned about long COVID

https://health.ucdavis.edu/news/headlines/11-things-doctors-have-learned-about-long-haul-covid/2022/02

30 - Macrophages, The Little Helpers That Heal Broken Blood Vessels

(VIDEO)

https://www.asianscientist.com/2016/05/in-the-lab/macrophages-microbleeds-heal-blood-vessels-neurodegenerative-diseases-cognitive-decline/

31 - How to Taper Antidepressants to Avoid a Withdrawal (Discontinuation) Syndrome? From, Dr Sanil Rege's Hub - Psychiatry Simplified

https://youtu.be/1wWCBPSj7ZA

32 - Distinguishing features of Long Covid identified through immune profiling

https://www.nature.com/articles/s41586-023-06651-y

33 - For These 17 COVID Long Haulers, Reactivated Viruses May Be to Blame

https://www.verywellhealth.com/long-covid-latent-viral-reactivations-5205269

34 - Herpes simplex Joseph E. Pizzorno ND, ...Herb Joiner-Bey ND, in The Clinician's Handbook of Natural Medicine (Third Edition), 2016

https://www.sciencedirect.com/topics/nursing-and-health-professions/herpes-simplex#:~:text=In%20herpes%20labialis%2C%20oral%20ascorbate,prevents%20disruption%20of%20vesicular%20membranes

35 - Quotes from EF Schumacher

https://centerforneweconomics.org/envision/legacy/ernst-friedrich-schumacher/small-is-beautiful-quotes/

36 - White Matter Hyperintensities on MRI - Coincidental Finding or Something Sinister? May 26, 2017 updated October 2, 2020

https://psychscenehub.com/psychinsights/white-matter-hyperintensities-mri/

37 - Nasal spray addiction: Is it real?

https://www.augustahealth.com/answer/nasal-spray-addiction-is-it-real/

38 - Can zero-calorie sweeteners raise your risk for cardiovascular disease?

https://www.medicalnewstoday.com/articles/can-zero-calorie-sweeteners-raise-your-risk-for-cardiovascular-disease

39 - Herpes medication and the COVID vaccines

https://herpes.org.uk/the-herpes-medication-and-the-covid-vaccines-it-is-ok/

40 - Covid-19 and Herpes Simplex Virus Infection: A Cross-Sectional Study

https://www.ncbi.nlm.nih.gov/pmc/articles/PMC8520410/

41 - Distinguishing features of Long Covid identified through immune profiling [cortisol finding]

https://www.medrxiv.org/content/10.1101/2022.08.09.22278592v1

42 - Guidance on "Long Covid" as a Disability Under the ADA, Section 504, and Section 1557

https://www.hhs.gov/civil-rights/for-providers/civil-rights-covid19/guidance-long-CoViD-disability/index.html

43 - Investigation of Long Covid Prevalence and Its Relationship to Epstein-Barr Virus Reactivation

https://www.ncbi.nlm.nih.gov/pmc/articles/PMC8233978/

44 - Covid-19 and Herpes Simplex Virus Infection: A Cross-Sectional Study

https://www.ncbi.nlm.nih.gov/pmc/articles/PMC8520410/

45 - Vitamin C May Be A Life Saver -

Mega-doses of Vitamin C can counter avian flu, hepatitis and herpes, and can even control the advance of Aids

https://www.independent.co.uk/life-style/health-and-families/health-news/vitamin-c-may-be-a-lifesaver-5544405.html

46 - According to Kaiser Pemanente

"...normally, cortisol levels rise during the early morning hours and are highest about 7 a.m. They drop very low in the evening and during the early phase of sleep. But if you sleep during the day and are up at night, this pattern may be reversed. If you do not have this daily change (diurnal rhythm) in cortisol levels, you may have overactive adrenal glands. This condition is called Cushing's syndrome."

https://wa.kaiserpermanente.org/kbase/topic.jhtml?docId=hw6227

47 - Can Antivirals Help in the Treatment of Long Covid?

https://www.medpagetoday.com/opinion/second-opinions/98570

48 - About VA Patient Advocates from VA website:

"There may come a time when you do not agree with your provider about the care that you are or will be receiving. Should this occur, discuss your concerns with your provider. If you still have concerns, ask to speak with your provider's supervisor or the Chief of the Service. If your concern is still unresolved, please contact the Patient Advocate who can assist you, if appropriate, in filing an appeal for a review of your concern."

https://www.va.gov/health/patientadvocate/

49 - Postural tachycardia syndrome (PoTS) - NHS

https://www.heart.org/en/news/2022/02/08/rehab-for-long-covid-gives-hope-while-condition-continues-to-puzzle'

50 - Long COVID's potentially 'devastating' impact on blood pressure

https://whyy.org/articles/the-unusual-relationship-between-covid-19-and-blood-pressure/

51 - Postural Orthostatic Tachycardia Syndrome (POTS)

https://my.clevelandclinic.org/health/diseases/16560-postural-orthostatic-tachycardia-syndrome-pots

52 - What doctors wish patients knew about long COVID

https://www.ama-assn.org/delivering-care/public-health/what-doctors-wish-patients-knew-about-long-covid

53 - The Importance of Listening in Treating Invisible Illness and Long-Haul COVID-19

https://journalofethics.ama-assn.org/article/importance-listening-treating-invisible-illness-and-long-haul-covid-19/2021-07

54 - Post-Acute COVID Syndrome (PACS)

https://covidprotocols.org/en/chapters/post-covid-care/

55 - Long COVID after breakthrough SARS-CoV-2 infection 25 May 2022

https://www.nature.com/articles/s41591-022-01840-0

56 - Can Antivirals Help in the Treatment of Long COVID?

https://www.medpagetoday.com/opinion/second-opinions/98570

57 - Valacyclovir (Oral Route) - uses of 2000mg for adults 2x daily for cold

sores

https://www.mayoclinic.org/drugs-supplements/Valacyclovir-oral-route/precautions/drg-20066635?p=1

58 - Detection of significant antiviral drug effects on COVID-19 with reasonable sample sizes in randomized controlled trials: A modeling study

https://journals.plos.org/plosmedicine/article?id=10.1371/journal.pmed.1003660

59 - Triangulating the truth, and how journalistic objectivity should work

https://beyondthetimes.com/2018/12/31/triangulating-the-truth-and-how-journalistic-objectivity-should-work/

60 - Management of post-acute covid-19 in primary care

https://www.bmj.com/content/370/bmj.m3026/infographic

61 - Long covid—an update for primary care

https://www.bmj.com/content/378/bmj-2022-072117

62 - Long COVID symptoms linked to inflammation

https://www.nih.gov/news-events/nih-research-matters/long-covid-symptoms-linked-inflammation

63 - From research above in ref# 61 - Benjamin tenOever, PhD, Professor, Department of Microbiology, Professor, Department of Medicine

https://med.nyu.edu/faculty/benjamin-tenoever Also: https://tenoeverlab.com/

64 - Caution advised with low histamine diets for Long Covid – Assoc. of UK Dietitians

https://www.bda.uk.com/resource/caution-advised-with-low-histamine-diets-for-long-covid.html

65 - Mental Health During the COVID-19 Pandemic - NIH

https://covid19.nih.gov/covid-19-topics/mental-health

66 - Why we need to keep using the patient made term "Long Covid"

https://blogs.bmj.com/bmj/2020/10/01/why-we-need-to-keep-using-the-patient-made-term-long-covid/

67 - Genital Herpes – CDC Detailed Fact Sheet

https://www.cdc.gov/std/herpes/stdfact-herpes-detailed.htm

68 - Long COVID or Post-COVID Conditions

https://www.cdc.gov/coronavirus/2019-ncov/long-term-effects/index.html

69 - Isolation and Precautions for People with COVID-19

https://www.cdc.gov/coronavirus/2019-ncov/your-health/isolation.html

70 - WHO launches new pandemic prevention plan, as COVID deaths fall 95 per cent

https://news.un.org/en/story/2023/04/1136052

71 - The latest long COVID research on symptoms, testing and treatments with Akiko Iwasaki, PhD

https://www.ama-assn.org/delivering-care/public-health/latest-long-covid-research-symptoms-testing-and-treatments-akiko

72 — Long COVID: What Do the Latest Data Show?

https://www.kff.org/policy-watch/long-covid-what-do-latest-data-show/

73 — Can Stimulating the Vagus Nerve Actually Transform Your Health?

https://www.verywellhealth.com/vagus-nerve-health-conditions-5219941

74 — In-Depth: Vagus nerve could control long COVID symptoms

https://www.10news.com/news/in-depth/in-depth-vagus-nerve-could-control-long-covid-symptoms

75 — Enhanced external counterpulsation for management of symptoms associated with long COVID

https://www.sciencedirect.com/science/article/pii/S2666602222000222

76 — Enhanced external counterpulsation for management of symptoms associated with long COVID (METHODOLOGY)

https://www.sciencedirect.com/science/article/pii/S2666602222000222#bb0015

77 — New Long COVID Findings Offer Fuller Picture of Condition

https://www.usnews.com/news/health-news/articles/2023-09-26/new-long-covid-findings-offer-fuller-picture-of-condition

78 — Large study provides scientists with deeper insight into long COVID symptoms

https://www.nih.gov/news-events/news-releases/large-study-provides-scientists-deeper-insight-into-long-covid-symptoms

79 — Long COVID and Significant Activity Limitation Among Adults, by Age — United States, June 1–13, 2022, to June 7–19, 2023

https://www.cdc.gov/mmwr/volumes/72/wr/mm7232a3.htm

80 — Long Covid symptoms ease for most within a year, new research finds

https://www.nbcnews.com/health/health-news/long-covid-symptoms-ease-year-new-research-finds-rcna65151

81 — A discovery in the muscles of long COVID patients may explain exercise troubles | Health News Florida

https://health.wusf.usf.edu/npr-health/2024-01-09/a-discovery-in-the-muscles-of-long-covid-patients-may-explain-exercise-troubles

82 — Muscle abnormalities worsen after post-exertional malaise in long COVID

https://www.nature.com/articles/s41467-023-44432-3

83 — Griffith RS, Norins AL, Kagan C. - A multicentered study of lysine therapy in Herpes simplex infection. - Dermatologica. 1978;156(5):257–267.

This multicenter clinical study examined oral L-lysine supplementation in patients with recurrent herpes simplex infection and reported reduced recurrence frequency and shortened healing time, consistent with proposed lysine–arginine competitive mechanisms affecting viral replication.

https://pubmed.ncbi.nlm.nih.gov/640102/

84 — Willow (Salix spp.) bark hot water extracts inhibit both enveloped and non-enveloped viruses: study on its anti-coronavirus and anti-enterovirus activities (2023)

https://converis.jyu.fi/converis/portal/detail/Publication/194520060?lang=en_GB

Personal Links

X (Twitter) JZ_Murdock: https://twitter.com/JZ_Murdock

YouTube: https://bit.ly/3uWwC1q

Amazon: https://amzn.to/2DEcS8u

Facebook: https://www.facebook.com/OfficialJZMurdock/

Personal Website: https://jzmurdock.com

Research Paper: "On Psychology: With Illustration in Psychopathology via Synesthesia and Schizophrenia"

On Amazon: https://www.amazon.com/gp/product/B008XCJ73I (also includes another paper: "Some Notes on Field Theory, Albert's Mind, Field Theory and the Statue Quo: The Necessity of Contextualism in Psychology"

Or on Smashwords: https://www.smashwords.com/books/view/209495

Film Production Website: http://lgnproductions.com

Films: Last good Nerve (LgN) Productions

I don't know how long these may be up online, but for what it's worth, here are interview links:

Interview: "Afternoons with Ash Black: JZ Murdock"

https://youtu.be/v0Lk4iVdyYg

https://vimeo.com/739770296

Also the interviews with my friends, two interesting guys who shot interviews that same day:

"Afternoons with Ash Black: Kelly Hughes" Director

https://youtu.be/Rhcp4JzMHt8

"Afternoons with Ash Black: Pat Moriarity" Cartoonist

https://youtu.be/E47wfCLjn4U

www.ingramcontent.com/pod-product-compliance
Lightning Source LLC
Chambersburg PA
CBHW051557250726
48653CB00004BA/1194